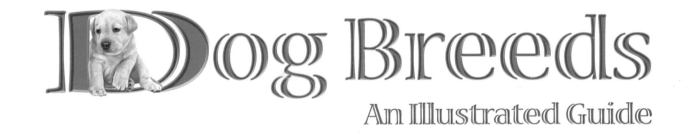

Dog Breeds

An Illustrated Guide

Anatomical Chart Company, Skokie, Illinois

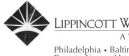

LIPPINCOTT WILLIAMS & WILKINS
A **Wolters Kluwer** Company

Philadelphia • Baltimore • New York • London
Buenos Aires • Hong Kong • Sydney • Tokyo

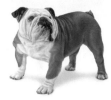

Published in the United States in 2002 by
The Anatomical Chart Company
A division of Lippincott Williams & Wilkins
A Wolters Kluwer Company
8221 Kimball Avenue,
Skokie, Illinois 60076-2956

First Edition

ISBN: 1-58779-480-2
Library of Congress Card Number: 2002102053

Anatomy consultant
M. S. A. Kumar, D.V.M., Ph.D.

Illustrations
Liana Bauman, M.A.M.S
Dawn Gorski, M.A.M.S
Lik Kwong, M.F.A.

Design
Urszula Adamowska, B.F.A.

Contributing writer
Dana Demas

Editor
Nancy Liskar

Production
Kassandra Porteous, B.F.A.

Printed and bound in the United States of America.

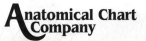

Anatomical Chart Company

CONTENTS

Skeletal Anatomy 4
- External Anatomy • Skeleton–Lateral View • Skeleton–Cranial View
- Skull *(lateral view and ventral view, mandible removed)*
- Left Carpus and Manus *(forepaw–palmar view)*
- Left Tarsus and Pes *(hindpaw–dorsal view, hindpaw–plantar view)*

Muscular Anatomy 10
- Muscular System *(lateral view)* • *Cranial view*
- Muscles of the Head *(superficial–lateral view, deep–lateral view)*

Systems & Organs 14
- The Organ Systems • The Respiratory System • Dorsal (Top) View of the Lungs
- The Digestive System • Ventral (Bottom) View of Abdominal Organs
- The Arterial Circulatory System • Left Lateral View of the Heart

Sporting Group 22
- Cocker Spaniel • Irish Setter • Labrador Retriever • Pointer
- Weimaraner

Hound Group 28
- Basset Hound • Beagle • Bloodhound • Dachshund • Greyhound

Terrier Group 34
- Airedale Terrier • Jack Russell Terrier • Kerry Blue Terrier
- Miniature Schnauzer • Scottish Terrier

Working Group 40
- Boxer • Doberman Pinscher • Great Dane • Saint Bernard • Siberian Husky

Non-Sporting Group 46
- Bichon Frise • Bulldog • Chow Chow • Dalmatian • Poodle

Toy Group 52
- Chihuahua • Japanese Chin • Pug • Shih Tzu • Yorkshire Terrier

Herding Group 58
- Australian Shepherd • Bouvier des Flandres • Collie
- German Shepherd Dog • Welsh Corgi (Pembroke)

**American Kennel Club
Recognized Breeds** 64

Credits 66

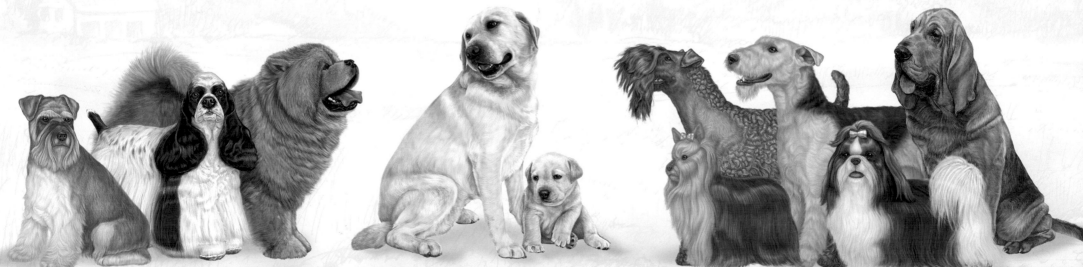

1

Skeletal Anatomy

The dog's skeleton serves as the structural framework for support and protection of the body. Along with muscles, the skeleton enables the dog to stand, sit, run, and walk.

Bones are hollow tubes made up of hard, latticed structures called trabeculae and are filled with bone marrow. Bones are nourished by blood vessels that enter them through small holes called nutrient foramina. Unlike humans, dogs do not have a collarbone; their forelimbs are held together by only the muscles. This allows dogs to have great flexibility in movement.

All dogs have 30 true vertebrae, plus a varying number found in the tail. The vertebrae are arranged in 5 groups: 7 cervical, 13 thoracic, 7 lumbar, 3 sacral, and the varying number of caudal (tail) vertebrae. The spinal cord lies within the vertebral canal in the spine for protection.

The canine skull comes in three basic shapes. The dolichocephalic shape, as seen in the Afghan Hound, is elongated and narrow. Short, broad heads, like that of the Bulldog, are called brachycephalic. Skulls of average length, like that of the Siberian Husky, are classified as mesocephalic.

External Anatomy

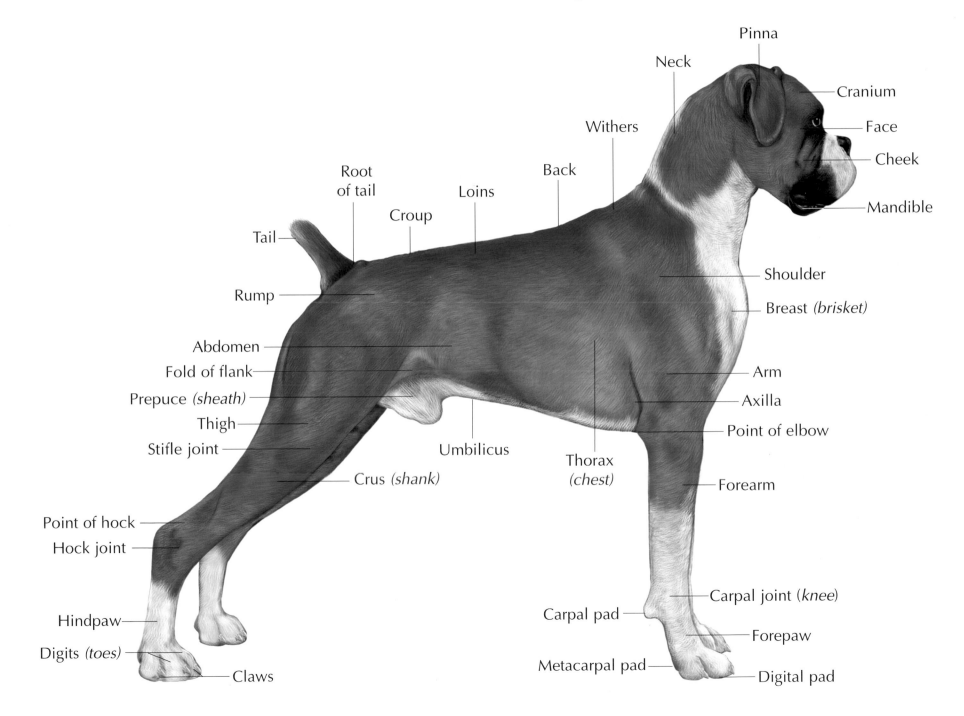

Pinna

Neck

Cranium

Withers

Face

Back

Cheek

Root of tail

Loins

Mandible

Croup

Tail

Shoulder

Rump

Breast *(brisket)*

Abdomen

Fold of flank

Arm

Prepuce *(sheath)*

Axilla

Thigh

Point of elbow

Stifle joint

Umbilicus

Crus *(shank)*

Thorax *(chest)*

Forearm

Point of hock

Hock joint

Carpal joint *(knee)*

Carpal pad

Hindpaw

Forepaw

Digits *(toes)*

Metacarpal pad

Claws

Digital pad

Skeleton-
Lateral view

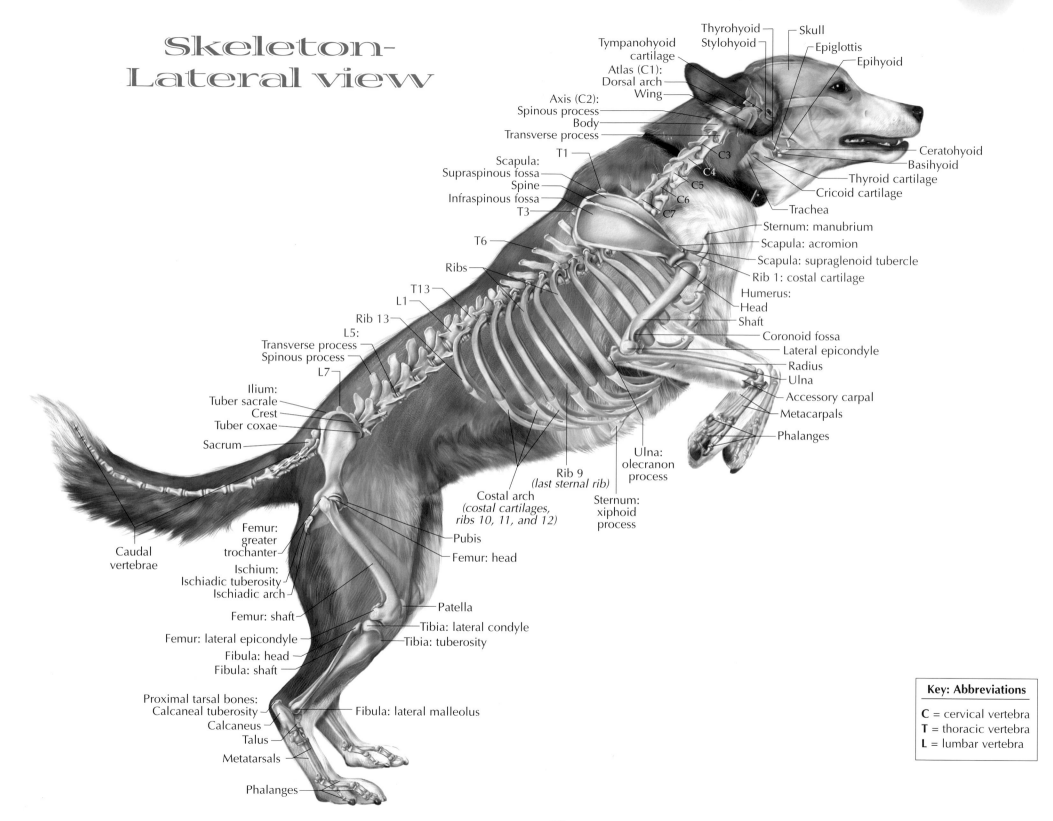

Thyrohyoid
Stylohyoid
Skull
Epiglottis
Epihyoid
Tympanohyoid cartilage
Atlas (C1):
Dorsal arch
Wing
Axis (C2):
Spinous process
Body
Transverse process
C3
C4
C5
C6
C7
T1
Scapula:
Supraspinous fossa
Spine
Infraspinous fossa
T3
T6
Ribs
T13
L1
Rib 13
L5:
Transverse process
Spinous process
L7
Ilium:
Tuber sacrale
Crest
Tuber coxae
Sacrum
Caudal vertebrae
Femur:
greater trochanter
Ischium:
Ischiadic tuberosity
Ischiadic arch
Femur: shaft
Femur: lateral epicondyle
Fibula: head
Fibula: shaft
Proximal tarsal bones:
Calcaneal tuberosity
Calcaneus
Talus
Metatarsals
Phalanges
Costal arch
(costal cartilages, ribs 10, 11, and 12)
Rib 9
(last sternal rib)
Pubis
Femur: head
Patella
Tibia: lateral condyle
Tibia: tuberosity
Fibula: lateral malleolus
Ulna: olecranon process
Sternum: xiphoid process
Ceratohyoid
Basihyoid
Thyroid cartilage
Cricoid cartilage
Trachea
Sternum: manubrium
Scapula: acromion
Scapula: supraglenoid tubercle
Rib 1: costal cartilage
Humerus:
Head
Shaft
Coronoid fossa
Lateral epicondyle
Radius
Ulna
Accessory carpal
Metacarpals
Phalanges

Key: Abbreviations

C = cervical vertebra
T = thoracic vertebra
L = lumbar vertebra

6

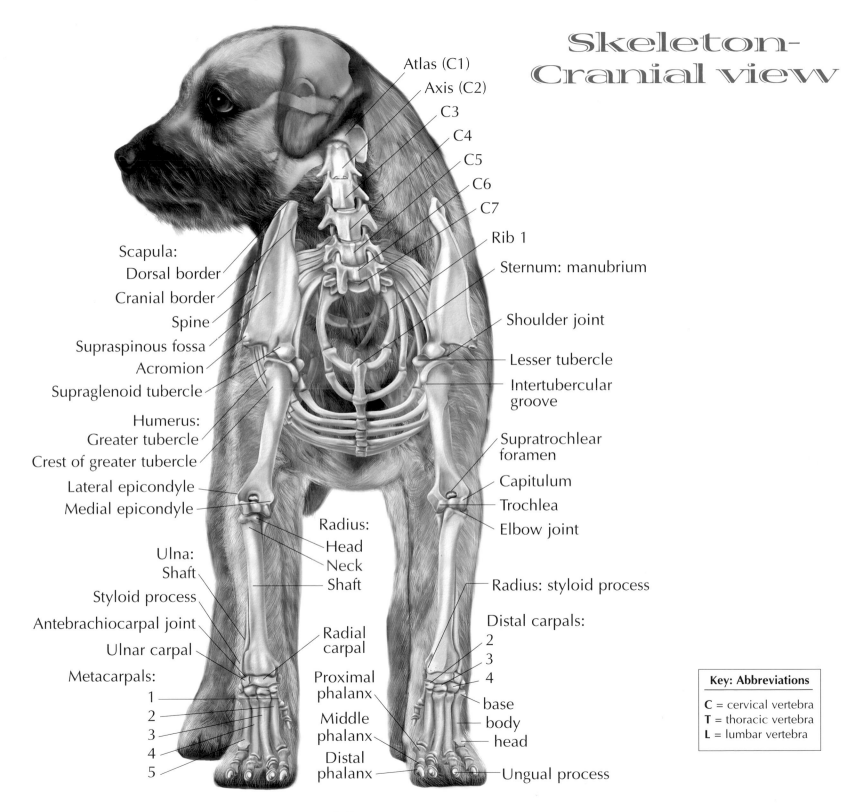

Atlas (C1)

Axis (C2)

C3

C4

C5

C6

C7

Rib 1

Sternum: manubrium

Scapula:

Dorsal border

Cranial border

Spine

Supraspinous fossa

Acromion

Supraglenoid tubercle

Humerus:
Greater tubercle

Crest of greater tubercle

Lateral epicondyle

Medial epicondyle

Shoulder joint

Lesser tubercle

Intertubercular
groove

Supratrochlear
foramen

Capitulum

Trochlea

Elbow joint

Radius:
Head
Neck
Shaft

Ulna:
Shaft

Styloid process

Antebrachiocarpal joint

Ulnar carpal

Radial
carpal

Radius: styloid process

Distal carpals:

2

3

4

base

body

head

Metacarpals:

1

2

3

4

5

Proximal
phalanx

Middle
phalanx

Distal
phalanx

Ungual process

Key: Abbreviations

C = cervical vertebra
T = thoracic vertebra
L = lumbar vertebra

Skull

Lateral view

Ventral view, mandible removed

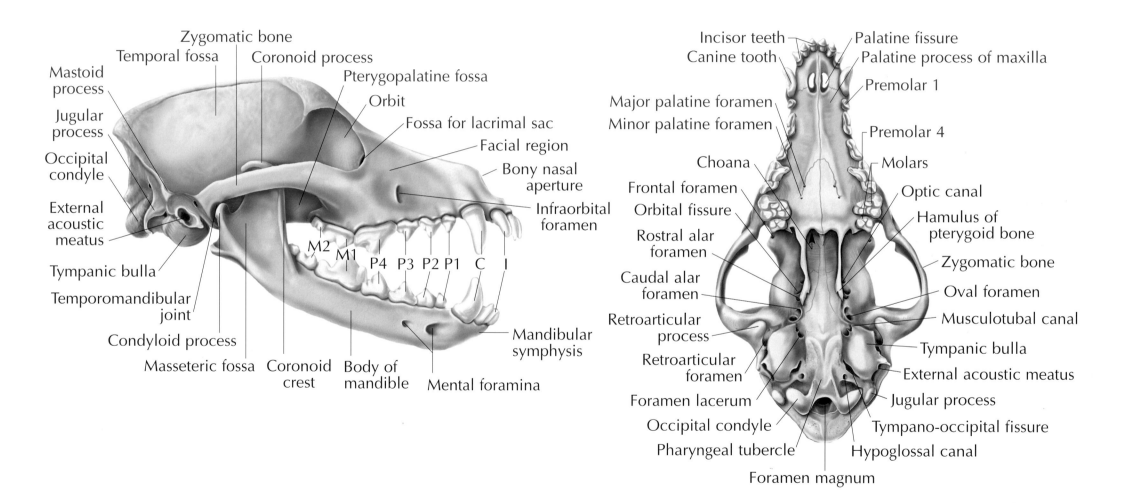

Lateral view labels:
Zygomatic bone
Temporal fossa
Coronoid process
Pterygopalatine fossa
Orbit
Fossa for lacrimal sac
Facial region
Bony nasal aperture
Infraorbital foramen
Mastoid process
Jugular process
Occipital condyle
External acoustic meatus
Tympanic bulla
Temporomandibular joint
Condyloid process
Masseteric fossa
Coronoid crest
Body of mandible
Mental foramina
Mandibular symphysis
M2 M1 P4 P3 P2 P1 C I

Ventral view labels:
Incisor teeth
Canine tooth
Palatine fissure
Palatine process of maxilla
Premolar 1
Major palatine foramen
Minor palatine foramen
Premolar 4
Molars
Choana
Optic canal
Frontal foramen
Orbital fissure
Hamulus of pterygoid bone
Rostral alar foramen
Zygomatic bone
Caudal alar foramen
Oval foramen
Retroarticular process
Musculotubal canal
Retroarticular foramen
Tympanic bulla
Foramen lacerum
External acoustic meatus
Occipital condyle
Jugular process
Pharyngeal tubercle
Tympano-occipital fissure
Hypoglossal canal
Foramen magnum

Key: Abbreviations

P = premolar teeth   **C** = canine teeth
I = incisor teeth   **M** = molar teeth

8

Left Carpus and Manus

Left Tarsus and Pes

Forepaw–palmar view

Hindpaw–dorsal view

Hindpaw–plantar view

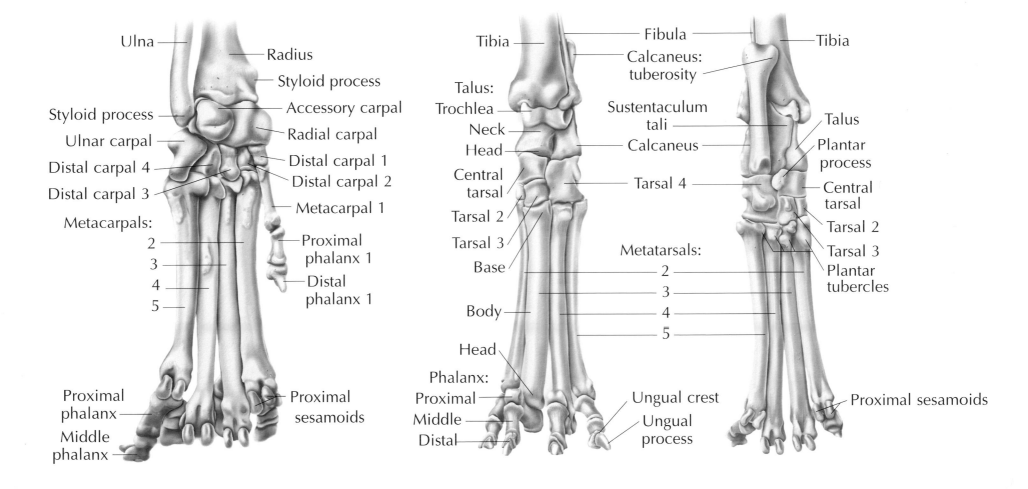

Ulna

Radius

Styloid process

Accessory carpal

Styloid process

Radial carpal

Ulnar carpal

Distal carpal 1

Distal carpal 4

Distal carpal 2

Distal carpal 3

Metacarpal 1

Metacarpals:

Proximal phalanx 1

2

3

Distal phalanx 1

4

5

Proximal phalanx

Proximal sesamoids

Middle phalanx

Tibia

Fibula

Tibia

Calcaneus: tuberosity

Talus:

Trochlea

Sustentaculum tali

Talus

Neck

Head

Calcaneus

Plantar process

Central tarsal

Tarsal 4

Central tarsal

Tarsal 2

Tarsal 3

Tarsal 2

Base

Metatarsals:

Tarsal 3

2

Plantar tubercles

3

Body

4

5

Head

Phalanx:

Proximal

Ungual crest

Middle

Ungual process

Distal

Proximal sesamoids

Muscular Anatomy

Muscles are necessary for movement, posture, breathing, circulation, and many other functions. Muscles also facilitate heat production to maintain body temperature. There are three types of muscles. Smooth muscle controls the movement of the large internal organs; cardiac muscle makes up most of the heart tissue. Striated, or skeletal, muscle makes up the rest of the muscle in the dog's body.

Skeletal muscle fibers are long, cylindrical, multi-nucleated cells organized into bundles; they are responsible for voluntary movement, that is, the dog can contract or relax the muscles at will. There are hundreds of skeletal muscles, each being a different size and shape and each having its own function. The ends of many skeletal muscles are attached to bones through fibrous, cordlike connective tissue called tendons. As muscle contracts, it moves one bone while another stays fairly stable. Skeletal muscles are arranged in layers that overlap each other. The muscles found just below the skin and fat are called superficial muscles; those found beneath the superficial muscles are called deep muscles.

Muscular System-
Lateral view

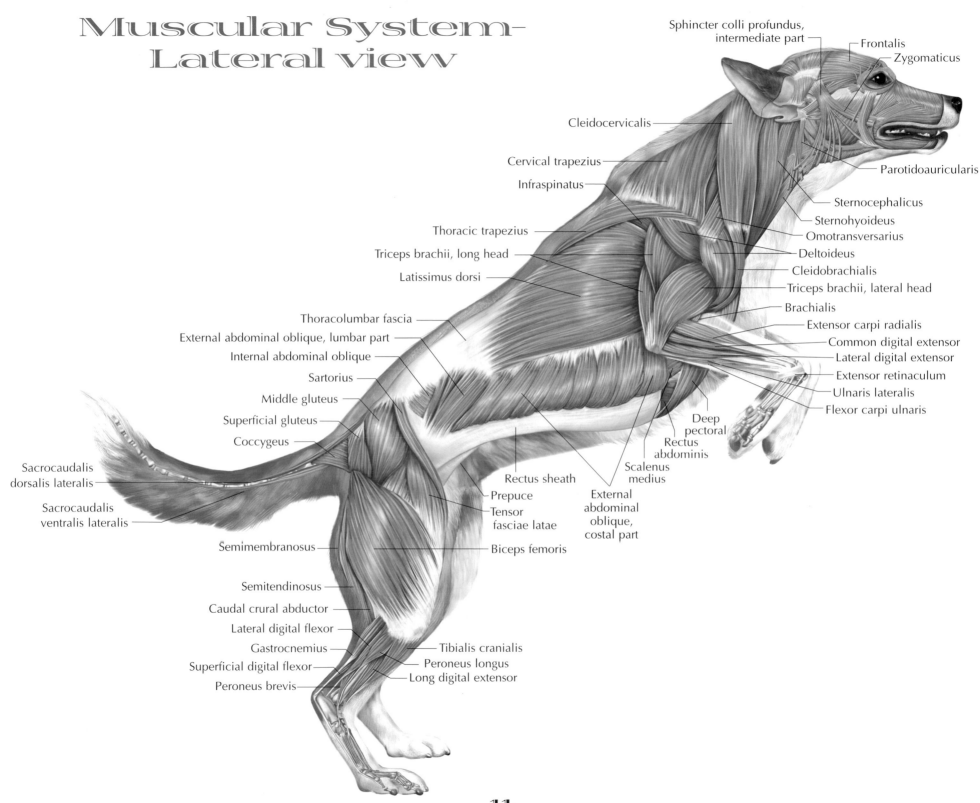

Sphincter colli profundus, intermediate part

Frontalis

Zygomaticus

Cleidocervicalis

Parotidoauricularis

Cervical trapezius

Infraspinatus

Sternocephalicus

Sternohyoideus

Thoracic trapezius

Omotransversarius

Triceps brachii, long head

Deltoideus

Latissimus dorsi

Cleidobrachialis

Triceps brachii, lateral head

Brachialis

Thoracolumbar fascia

Extensor carpi radialis

External abdominal oblique, lumbar part

Common digital extensor

Internal abdominal oblique

Lateral digital extensor

Sartorius

Extensor retinaculum

Middle gluteus

Ulnaris lateralis

Superficial gluteus

Flexor carpi ulnaris

Coccygeus

Deep pectoral

Rectus abdominis

Sacrocaudalis dorsalis lateralis

Scalenus medius

Rectus sheath

Sacrocaudalis ventralis lateralis

Prepuce

Tensor fasciae latae

External abdominal oblique, costal part

Semimembranosus

Biceps femoris

Semitendinosus

Caudal crural abductor

Lateral digital flexor

Gastrocnemius

Tibialis cranialis

Peroneus longus

Superficial digital flexor

Long digital extensor

Peroneus brevis

11

Cranial View

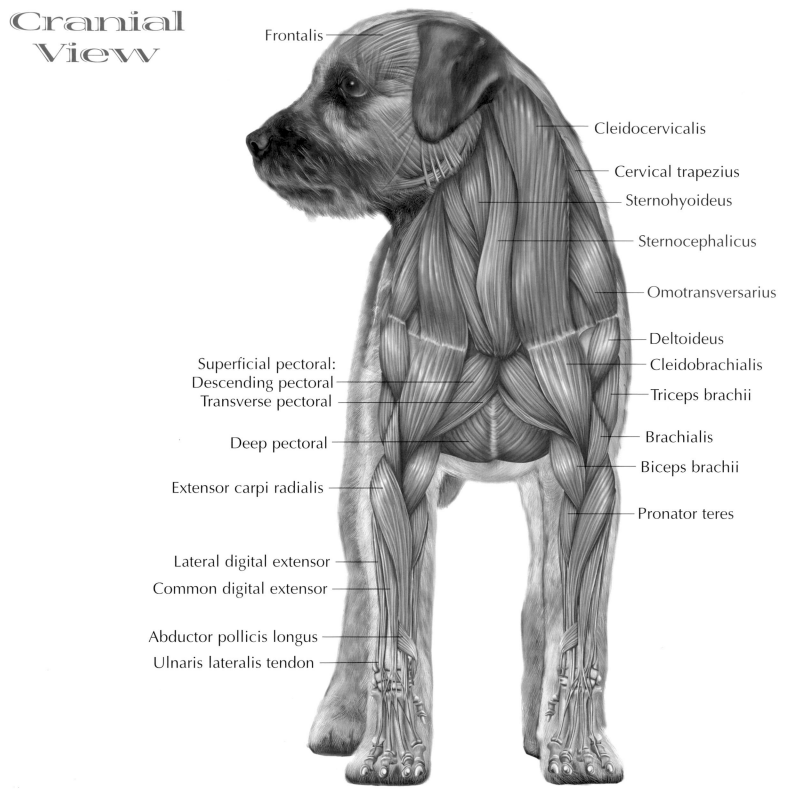

Frontalis

Cleidocervicalis

Cervical trapezius

Sternohyoideus

Sternocephalicus

Omotransversarius

Deltoideus

Superficial pectoral:

Descending pectoral

Cleidobrachialis

Transverse pectoral

Triceps brachii

Brachialis

Deep pectoral

Biceps brachii

Extensor carpi radialis

Pronator teres

Lateral digital extensor

Common digital extensor

Abductor pollicis longus

Ulnaris lateralis tendon

Muscles of the Head

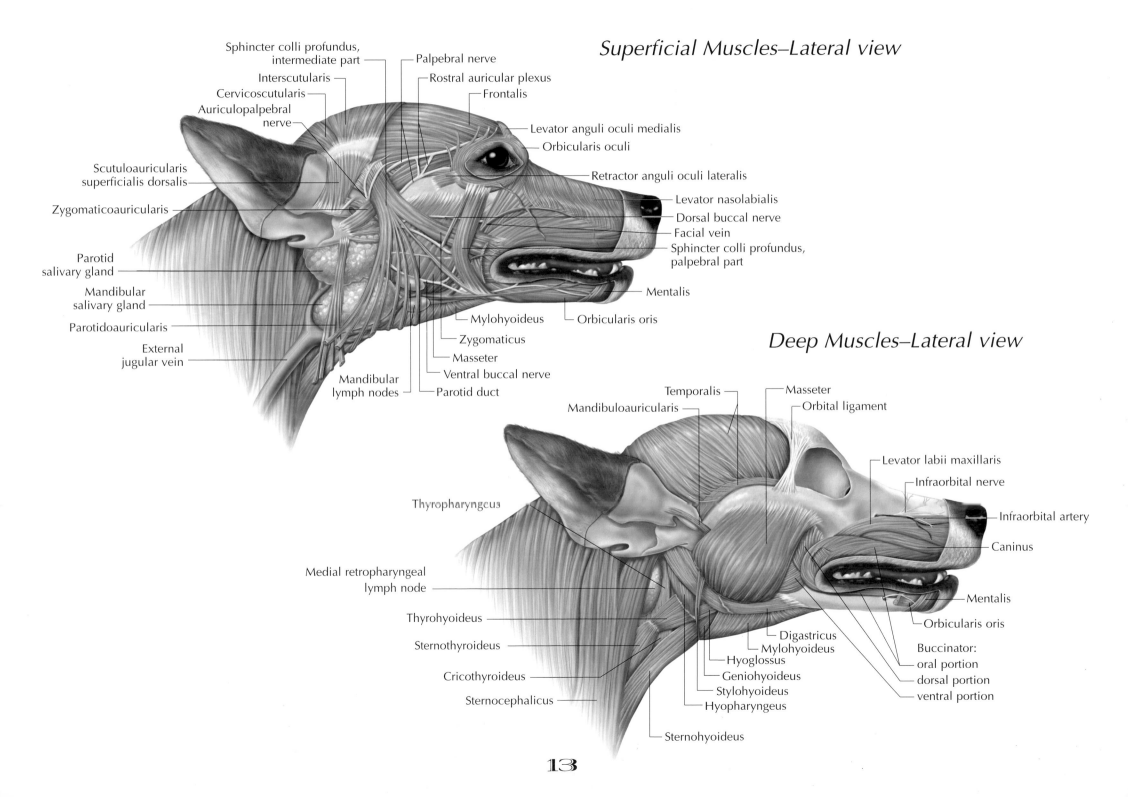

Superficial Muscles–Lateral view

Sphincter colli profundus, intermediate part
Interscutularis
Cervicoscutularis
Auriculopalpebral nerve
Palpebral nerve
Rostral auricular plexus
Frontalis
Levator anguli oculi medialis
Orbicularis oculi
Scutuloauricularis superficialis dorsalis
Retractor anguli oculi lateralis
Zygomaticoauricularis
Levator nasolabialis
Dorsal buccal nerve
Facial vein
Sphincter colli profundus, palpebral part
Parotid salivary gland
Mandibular salivary gland
Parotidoauricularis
External jugular vein
Mentalis
Mylohyoideus
Orbicularis oris
Zygomaticus
Masseter
Ventral buccal nerve
Mandibular lymph nodes
Parotid duct

Deep Muscles–Lateral view

Temporalis
Mandibuloauricularis
Masseter
Orbital ligament
Levator labii maxillaris
Infraorbital nerve
Infraorbital artery
Thyropharyngeus
Caninus
Medial retropharyngeal lymph node
Mentalis
Thyrohyoideus
Orbicularis oris
Sternothyroideus
Digastricus
Mylohyoideus
Buccinator:
oral portion
dorsal portion
ventral portion
Cricothyroideus
Hyoglossus
Geniohyoideus
Stylohyoideus
Sternocephalicus
Hyopharyngeus
Sternohyoideus

13

Systems & Organs

The dog's anatomy and physiology make it adaptable to its varied environment. This is possible only if all of the systems work together to maintain a healthy dog.

The circulatory system works to supply oxygen and other forms of energy to all parts of the body. When a dog is exercising, circulation (blood flow) accelerates dramatically: The blood flow to the heart's muscles increases fourfold, and the blood flow to the rest of the body increases 20 times more.

The respiratory system, which consists of air passages, lungs, and breathing muscles, works to provide fresh oxygen to the circulatory system. A considerable amount of oxygen is essential when a dog is active. By working together, the circulatory and respiratory systems produce enough energy to sustain the dog's active lifestyle.

A dog's digestive system works to break down food in the mouth, stomach, and intestines. Once the food is broken down, the body can easily process and use it as energy for the growth and repair of organs and tissues.

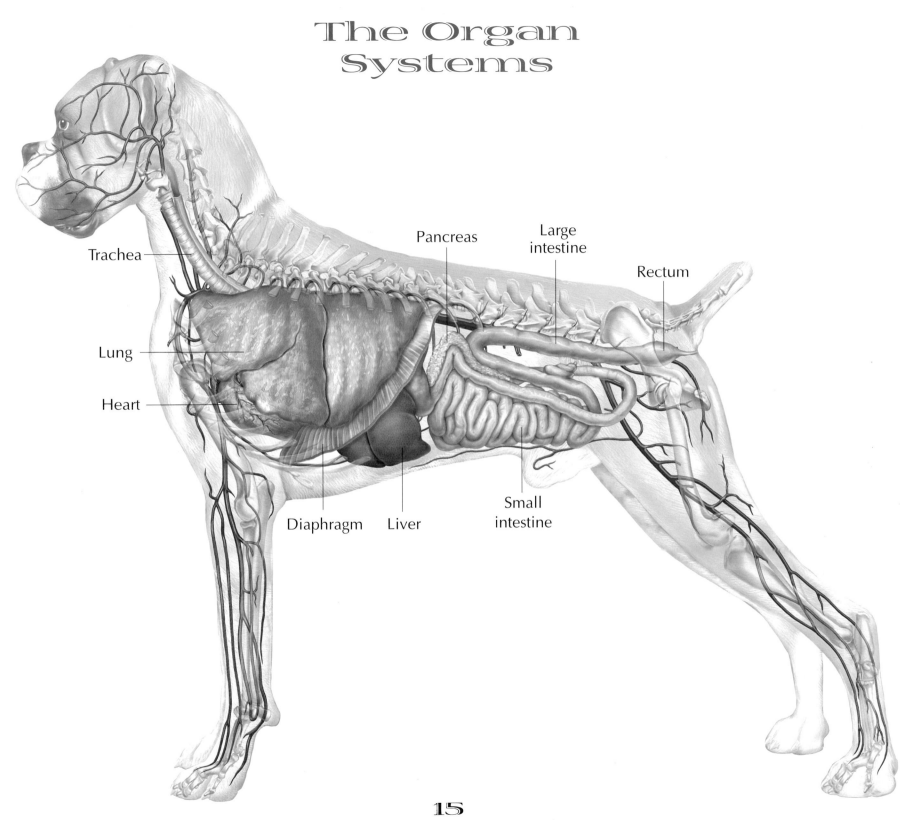

Trachea

Pancreas

Large intestine

Rectum

Lung

Heart

Diaphragm

Liver

Small intestine

The Respiratory System

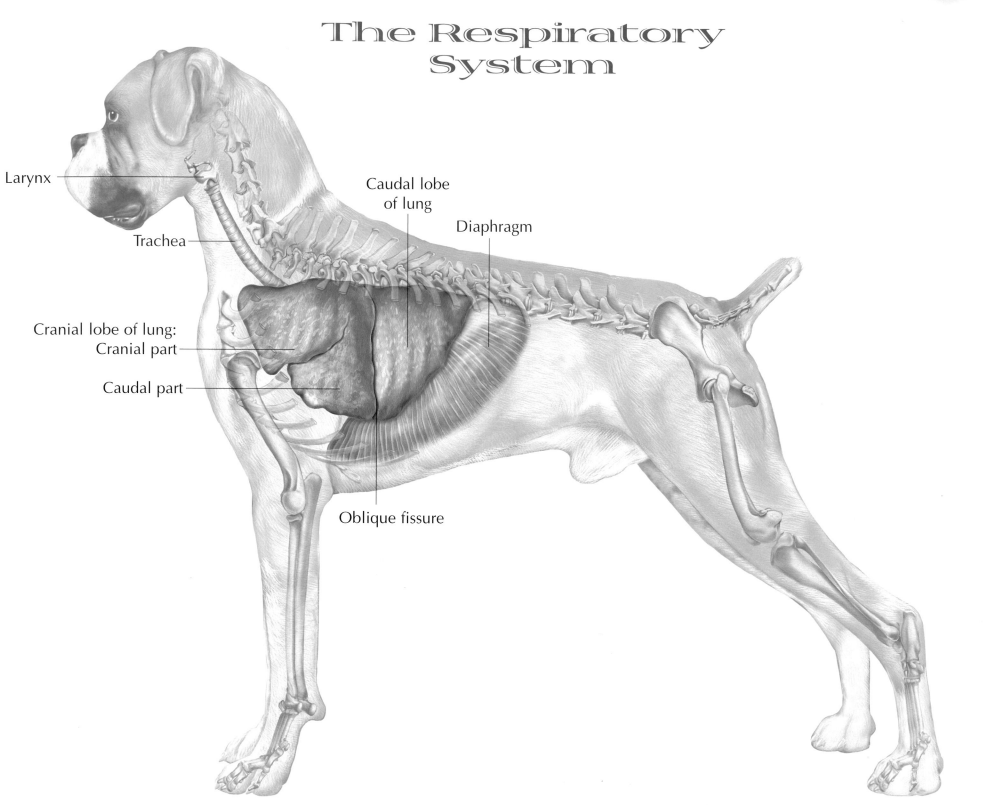

Larynx

Trachea

Caudal lobe of lung

Diaphragm

Cranial lobe of lung:

Cranial part

Caudal part

Oblique fissure

Dorsal (Top) View
of the Lungs

Left   *Right*

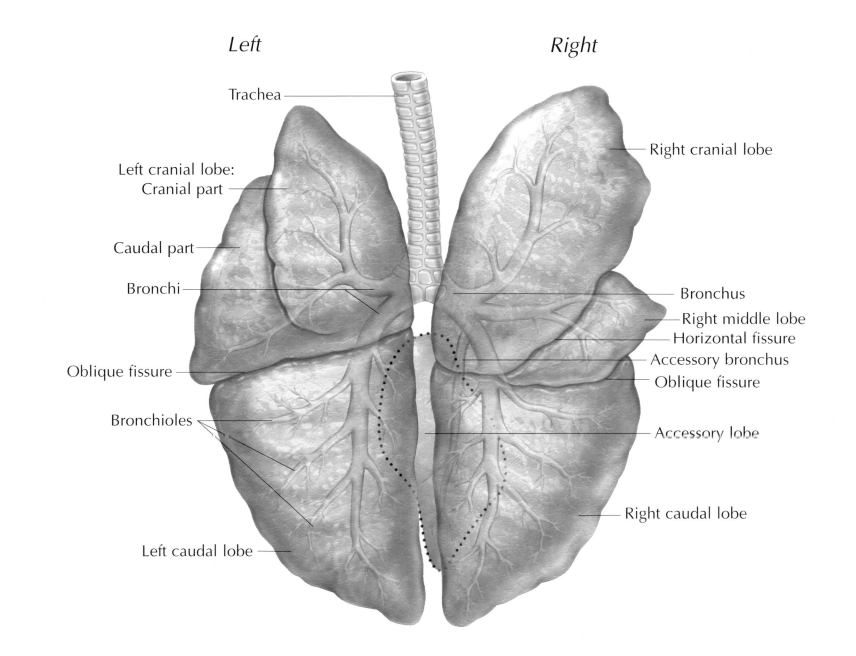

Trachea

Left cranial lobe:
Cranial part

Caudal part

Bronchi

Oblique fissure

Bronchioles

Left caudal lobe

Right cranial lobe

Bronchus

Right middle lobe

Horizontal fissure

Accessory bronchus

Oblique fissure

Accessory lobe

Right caudal lobe

The Digestive System

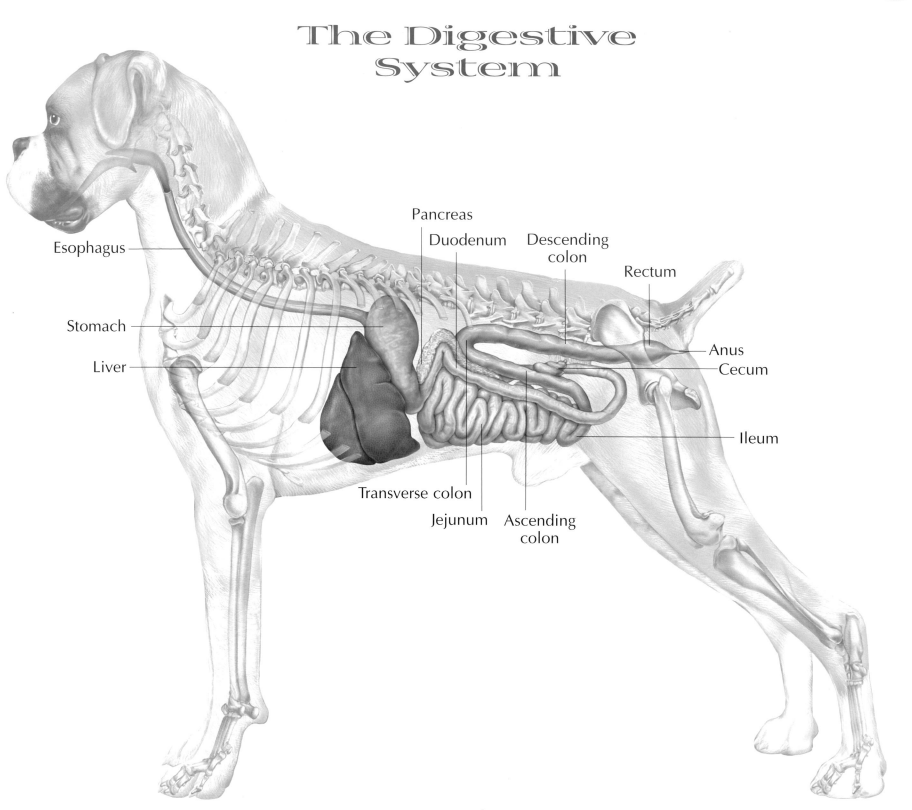

Esophagus

Stomach

Liver

Pancreas

Duodenum

Descending colon

Rectum

Anus

Cecum

Ileum

Transverse colon

Jejunum

Ascending colon

Ventral (Bottom) View of Abdominal Organs

Right   *Left*

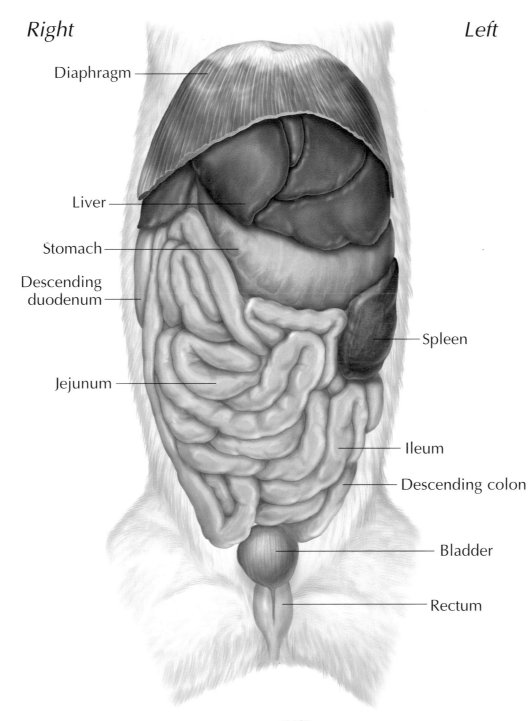

Diaphragm

Liver

Stomach

Descending
duodenum

Jejunum

Spleen

Ileum

Descending colon

Bladder

Rectum

The Arterial Circulatory System

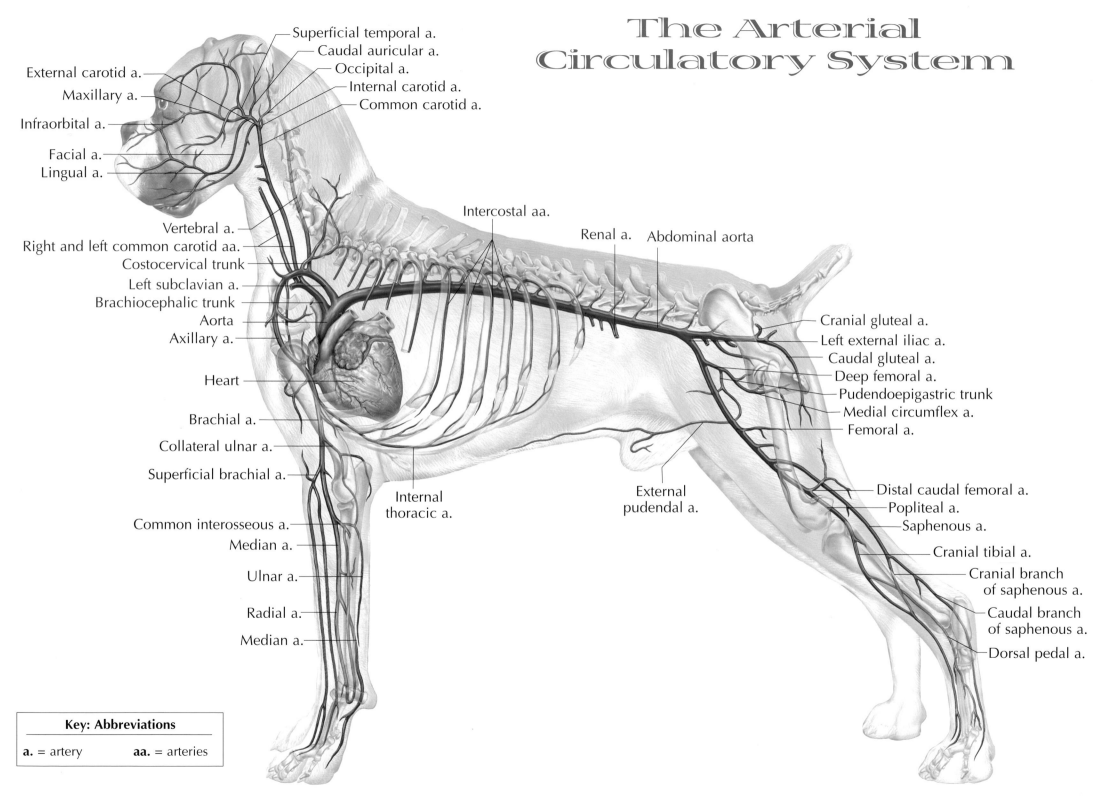

Superficial temporal a.
Caudal auricular a.
Occipital a.
Internal carotid a.
Common carotid a.

External carotid a.
Maxillary a.
Infraorbital a.
Facial a.
Lingual a.

Vertebral a.
Right and left common carotid aa.
Costocervical trunk
Left subclavian a.
Brachiocephalic trunk
Aorta
Axillary a.

Heart

Brachial a.
Collateral ulnar a.
Superficial brachial a.

Common interosseous a.
Median a.
Ulnar a.
Radial a.
Median a.

Intercostal aa.

Renal a.   Abdominal aorta

Internal
thoracic a.

External
pudendal a.

Cranial gluteal a.
Left external iliac a.
Caudal gluteal a.
Deep femoral a.
Pudendoepigastric trunk
Medial circumflex a.
Femoral a.

Distal caudal femoral a.
Popliteal a.
Saphenous a.
Cranial tibial a.
Cranial branch of saphenous a.
Caudal branch of saphenous a.
Dorsal pedal a.

Key: Abbreviations

a. = artery   **aa.** = arteries

Left Lateral View of the Heart

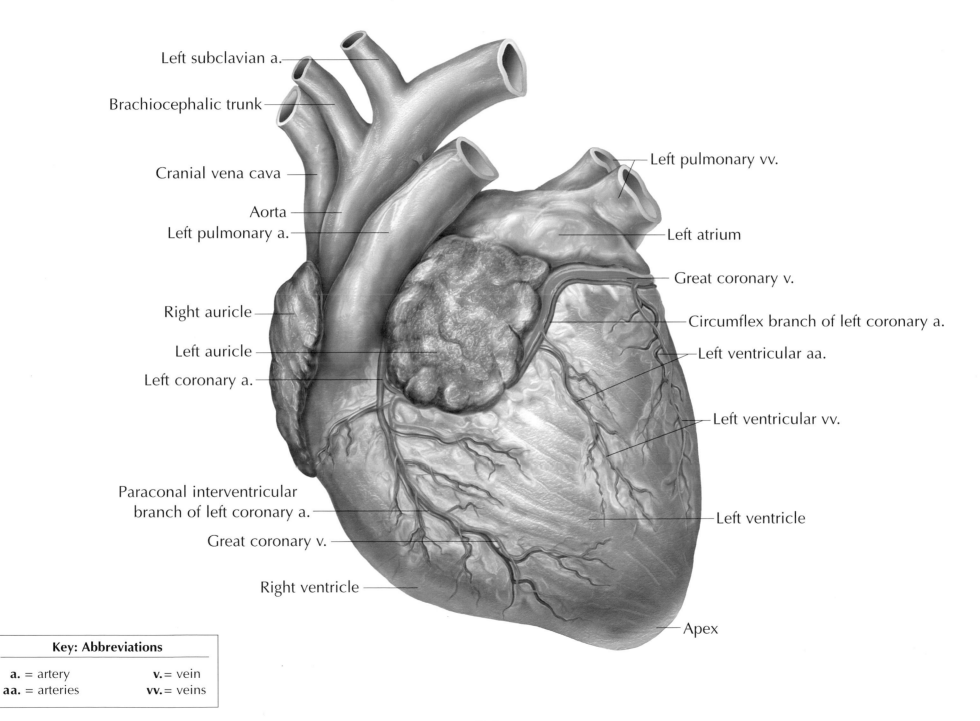

Left subclavian a.

Brachiocephalic trunk

Cranial vena cava

Aorta

Left pulmonary a.

Right auricle

Left auricle

Left coronary a.

Paraconal interventricular branch of left coronary a.

Great coronary v.

Right ventricle

Left pulmonary vv.

Left atrium

Great coronary v.

Circumflex branch of left coronary a.

Left ventricular aa.

Left ventricular vv.

Left ventricle

Apex

Key: Abbreviations	
a. = artery	**v.** = vein
aa. = arteries	**vv.** = veins

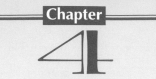

Sporting Group

By far the best known of all the groups, the sporting dogs are talented in the outdoors and warmly loved in millions of American households. This group was developed several centuries ago to help hunters in their pursuit of prey. Some breeds demonstrate the exceptional ability to track prey and then "point" or "freeze," indicating to hunters the location of quarry. Others assist by flushing out and then retrieving birds from the water, land, or marshes. On the whole, they are well suited to domestic life, but their exercise needs are great and should be considered in deciding whether to adopt these dogs as pets. Sporting dogs enjoy participating in activities they were bred for, such as swimming and retrieving—and an object as simple as a tennis ball or Frisbee will do perfectly. Sporting dogs are smart and energetic, and their endearing temperament and love of people make them ideal as family pets.

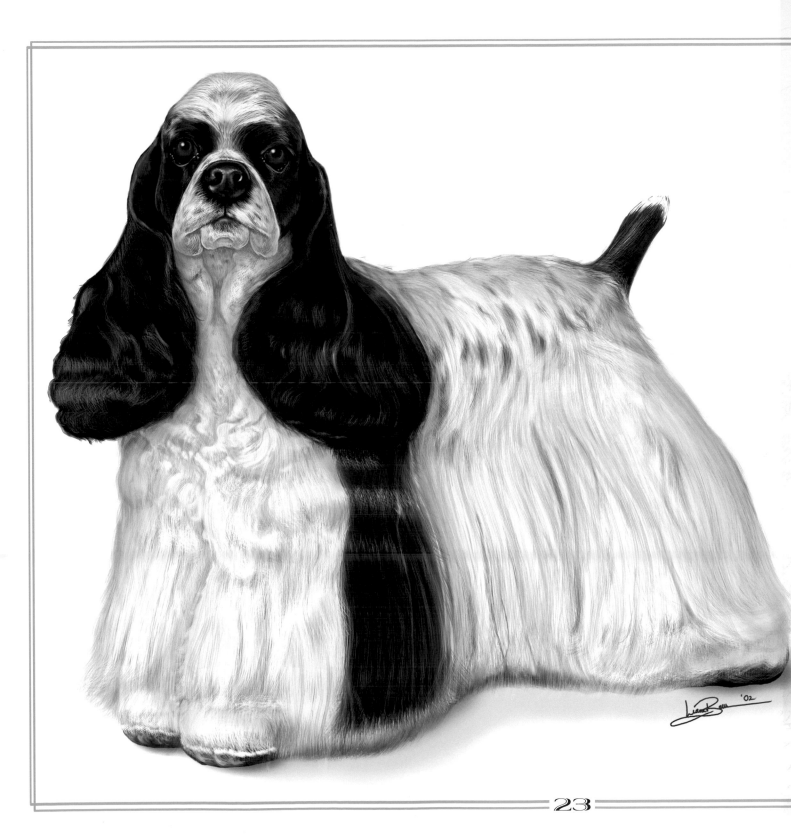

Cocker Spaniel

The adaptable and affectionate Cocker Spaniel is the smallest of the sporting dogs. Descended from the English Cocker Spaniel, the American breed was developed in the 19th century to flush out and retrieve quail. The American Cocker Spaniel has gone on to become a favorite family pet, as it can adjust to nearly any living situation and truly adores master and children alike.

The American Cocker Spaniel has a beautiful, silky coat that can be flat or slightly wavy. Colors range from black to red to white—and everything in between. Grooming this breed is somewhat demanding and involves brushing and combing several times a week, plus trimming every couple of months.

The companionable American Cocker Spaniel is a great family dog that is eager to please and easy to train. It is admired for its lively, intelligent personality and people-loving behavior— especially around children. The American Cocker Spaniel needs adequate exercise to avoid becoming overweight.

Height . . . . 13–15 in. / 34–39 cm
Weight . . . . 24–28 lb / 11–13 kg
Grooming . . . . high
Exercise . . . . medium
Appetite . . . . low
Lifespan . . . . 12–15 years

Irish Setter

Highly energetic and friendly to the core, the Irish Setter is believed to have originated in Ireland in the 1700s. The Irish Setter was bred to hunt birds, identifying the location of prey for hunters by sitting down. This outgoing, effervescent dog loves to play and run and usually lives a long, hearty life.

The Irish Setter is most recognizable by its coat, which is a shiny, deep mahogany red, feathering around the ears and across the underside and legs. Brushing and combing several days a week and trimming every three months are necessary to keep the coat in top condition.

Irish Setters enjoy interacting with people, children, and other animals, proving them to be among the most sociable of dogs. Obedience training should begin early in life to engage the Irish Setter's attention, as this breed has a tendency to become distracted. Irish Setters require ample exercise and room to run free. They generally do not make good watchdogs due to their friendly nature.

Height . . . . 25–27 in. / 63–69 cm
Weight . . . . 60–70 lb / 27–32 kg
Grooming . . . . medium
Exercise . . . . high
Appetite . . . . medium
Lifespan . . . . 12–14 years

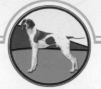

Labrador Retriever

By far Americans' favorite breed, the Labrador Retriever excels as both a sporting dog and a family pet. The Labrador originated in 19th-century Newfoundland, where it was used to retrieve and bring to shore the nets used by local fishermen. Despite the Labrador's current cult-like status as a household pet, this talented breed remains a skilled hunter and is frequently used as a bomb-sniffing dog, police dog, and guide dog for the visually impaired.

The Labrador's coat is nearly weatherproof, consisting of a short, dense outercoat and soft, insulating undercoat. Coat colors are black, yellow, or—more rarely—chocolate. A quick brushing once a week is the only grooming needed.

It is no surprise that the Labrador is such a fixture in American households. Gentle and loving, Labradors are easy to train, make excellent guard dogs, and love playing with children. Daily exercise is essential, especially given the Labrador's tendency to overeat and become sedentary. Playtime that involves swimming and retrieving, as often as possible, is highly recommended.

Height	21–24 in. / 55–62 cm
Weight	55–80 lb / 25–36 kg
Grooming	low
Exercise	medium
Appetite	medium
Lifespan	10–12 years

Pointer

The Pointer is named for its remarkable ability to reveal the location of prey to a hunter by raising one of its paws and remaining completely motionless. Normally used to hunt birds, Pointers display exceptional stamina and passion. The breed's exact origins are unclear, though it is known to have enjoyed popularity more than 300 years ago in England. The Pointer is an intelligent, active dog that needs lots of exercise.

The Pointer's coat is short and dense; colors include liver, lemon, black, or orange, all usually combined with white. Grooming requires a quick brushing to remove dead hair.

Pointers can be sensitive and easily distracted from everyday matters, necessitating early and thorough obedience training. Given their penchant for hunting, Pointers need vigorous exercise and activities to put their energy into, such as retrieving. They also enjoy learning new things and excel at competitive endeavors. Pointers are gentle with youngsters but may be too energetic at times for very small children.

Height	23–28 in. / 58–71 cm
Weight	44–75 lb / 20–34 kg
Grooming	low
Exercise	high
Appetite	high
Lifespan	12–15 years

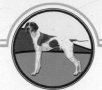

Weimaraner

Nicknamed the "gray ghost" for its distinctive gray coat, the Weimaraner's exact origins are also something of a shadow. This regal-looking breed is thought to date back to 19th-century Germany, where the ruling family is said to have favored it. Whatever its history, the Weimaraner is renowned for its skillfulness as a fast and reliable hunter, able to track and retrieve large game using its excellent sense of smell.

The Weimaraner's shiny coat can be any of several shades of gray, ranging from mouse-gray to silver-gray. Grooming the short, straight coat is simple—one quick brushing a week will do. Weimaraners have distinctive blue or amber-colored eyes that add to their unique appeal.

The talented Weimaraner likes to hunt and performs well with its master. It is a smart dog, however, and can be resistant to training if not handled firmly from early in life. Weimaraners are good with youngsters but sometimes can be a little too bold and rambunctious for small children. They also make excellent watchdogs. They require a lot of activity to avoid behavior problems.

Height . . . . 23–27 in. / 58–68cm
Weight . . . . 70–85 lb /32–38 kg
Grooming. . . . . low
Exercise . . . . high
Appetite. . . . . medium
Lifespan . . . . 10–13 years

5

Hound Group

Hounds were literally born to hunt, either by scent or by sight, many thousands of years ago. They have been used throughout history to track animals, people, and even lost treasure! Based on the faculty they use, hounds are unofficially grouped into two categories: scent hounds and gazehounds. Designed to hunt and not to kill, hounds were the first dogs to be trained and put to use by human beings. They are surprisingly not vicious and use their keen senses only to chase and isolate their prey, leaving the killing to their human counterparts. Despite their common skill in hunting, the hounds are a diverse group. On the whole, they make excellent house pets—but even the most domesticated of them may wander in pursuit of prey, making a fenced-in yard a necessity. Potential owners also should be prepared for the distinctive sound of baying, a habit that most hounds share.

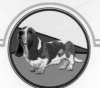

Basset Hound

Descended from the Bloodhound, the Basset Hound uses its remarkable sense of smell to hunt rabbits, foxes, and hares. It was bred in 16th-century France and is second only to the Bloodhound in its scent-driven tracking. The Basset Hound is a gracious dog that gets along superbly with other dogs and children.

The Basset Hound is best known for its long ears and droopy eyes, the most notable features of its sad but sweet face. Its coat is short, hard, and glossy and can be virtually any color. A rather large dog on very short legs, the Basset Hound needs only an occasional bathing. Weekly brushing and ear cleaning are also necessary.

Basset Hounds, which can be stubborn and challenging to housebreak, require early obedience training. They need regular exercise and controlled food intake so they do not become heavy. Truly loving dogs, Basset Hounds do not become destructive if left alone. When they are not fenced in, they should always be kept on a leash to prevent them from wandering off.

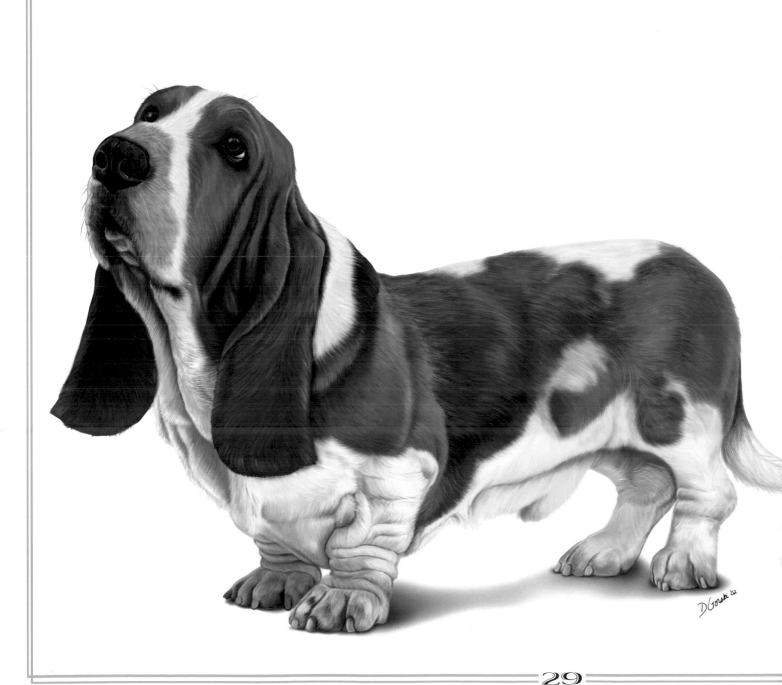

Height . . . . 13–15 in. / 33–38 cm
Weight. . . . . 40–60 lb / 18–27 kg
Grooming . . . . medium
Exercise . . . . medium
Appetite. . . . . high
Lifespan . . . . 10–13 years

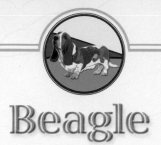

Beagle

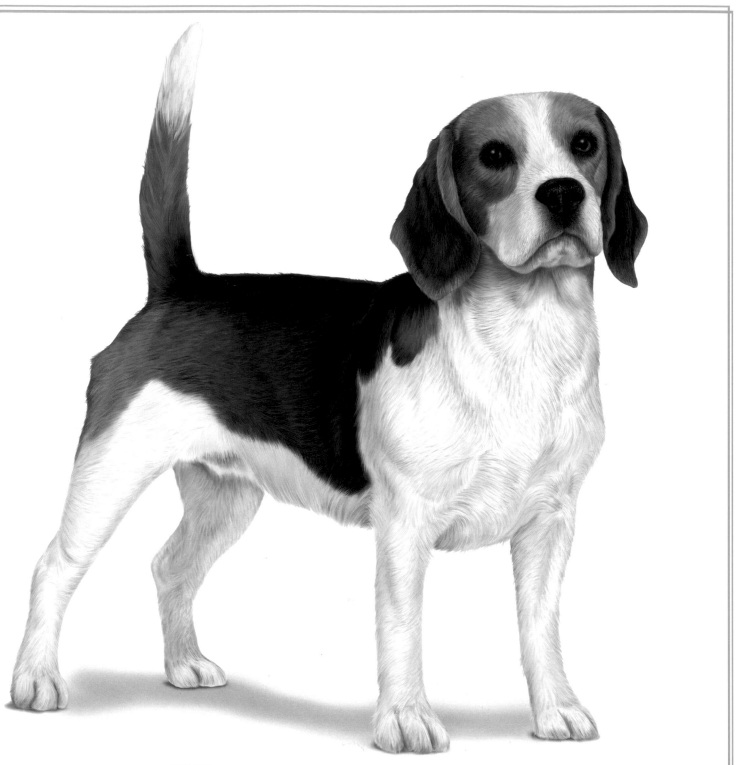

A lovable little rascal, the Beagle is the smallest member of the hound group and was bred as far back as the 14th century to chase and hunt hare and pheasant. Beagles are most at home in a pack, making them friendly dogs that enjoy the company of children and other dogs. Mischievous but irresistible, the Beagle has become a popular household pet.

Beagles can be found in almost any color, usually displaying some combination of white, tan, and black. Their coats can be rough or smooth and require very little grooming. By nature, Beagles are clean dogs that do not drool or have an unpleasant body odor.

Notorious for their wandering, Beagles should not be allowed to roam unsupervised unless confined to a safely fenced yard. Beagles should also begin obedience training early to help curtail habits like digging and excessive barking. Beagles are gentle dogs that do well with children and other dogs. They make good watchdogs and have a pleasing howl.

Height . . . . 12–15 in. / 30–38 cm
Weight . . . . 18–30 lb / 8–14 kg
Grooming . . . . low
Exercise . . . . medium
Appetite . . . . medium
Lifespan . . . . 12–15 years

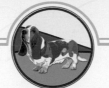

Bloodhound

The genial Bloodhound is thought to have originated in ancient Greece or Italy, with the modern type developed about one thousand years ago in England. Like the best of the scent-tracking hounds, the Bloodhound has an impressive history as a police dog. The Bloodhound is used to track missing people and animals, lost possessions, and trails that are often days old. Its superb sense of smell is matched only by its gentle nature and placid demeanor.

The Bloodhound's unique face is marked by a generous amount of sagging skin, droopy eyes, and long ears that help it to capture scent. Its coat is short and smooth; colors include black and tan, red and tan, and tawny. Weekly brushing and ear cleaning are needed.

Though a great hunter, like other hounds the Bloodhound does not have the killer instinct. It gets along exceptionally well with other dogs and children. Although Bloodhounds are quick to learn, stubbornness is a problem when it comes to obedience training, which makes early training essential. Bloodhounds need plenty of daily exercise and should be fed smaller meals several times a day, as they are voracious eaters.

Height	23–27 in. / 58–68 cm
Weight	80–110 lb /36–50 kg
Grooming	low
Exercise	high
Appetite	high
Lifespan	8–10 years

Dachshund

The Dachshund was bred in 16th-century Germany to hunt badgers. The result of a hound-terrier crossbreed, the Dachshund is like a terrier in that it will burrow into the ground in pursuit of a badger or other small animal. Its low-to-the-ground, elongated shape allows it to slip in and out of holes easily. Spirited and bright, the Dachshund has become a popular house pet due to its pleasant disposition and usefulness as a watchdog.

Dachshunds come in two sizes, standard and miniature, and can be smooth, long, or wire-haired, making for six distinct varieties. Coat colors for all types include black, brindle, gray, chocolate, fawn, and white with tan or black markings. Grooming smooth and wire-haired varieties requires occasional brushing. Longhaired varieties need brushing every other day.

Though affable, Dachshunds are stubborn and need early obedience training. They enjoy children and other dogs, but they tend to be wary of strangers. Dachshunds' exercise needs are low, but their weight should be monitored. Dachshunds are companionable dogs that most enjoy relaxing with those they know.

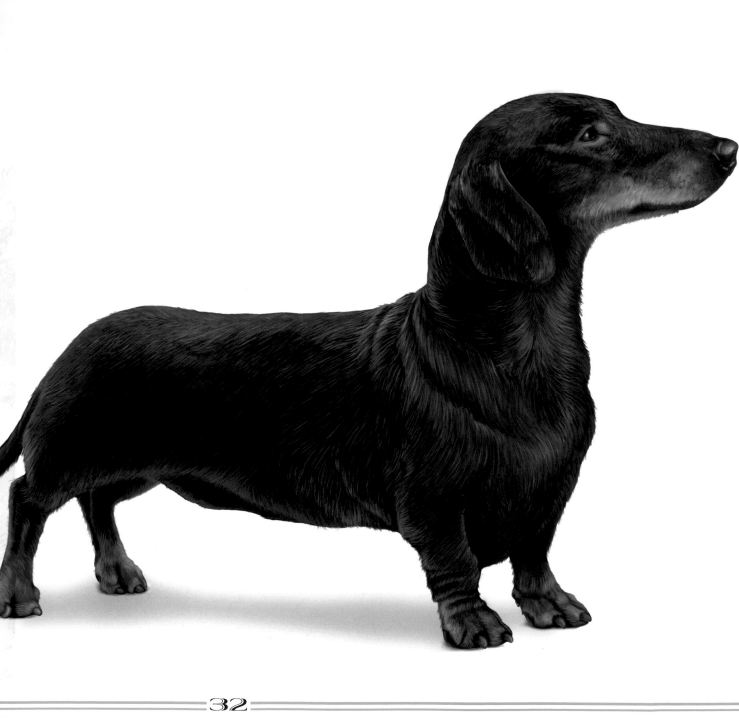

Height	Standard	9–10 in. / 23–25 cm
	Miniature	5–9 in. / 13–23 cm
Weight	Standard	16–32 lb / 7–14 kg
	Miniature	9–10 lb / 4–5 kg
Grooming		low
Exercise		low
Appetite		low
Lifespan		12–15 years

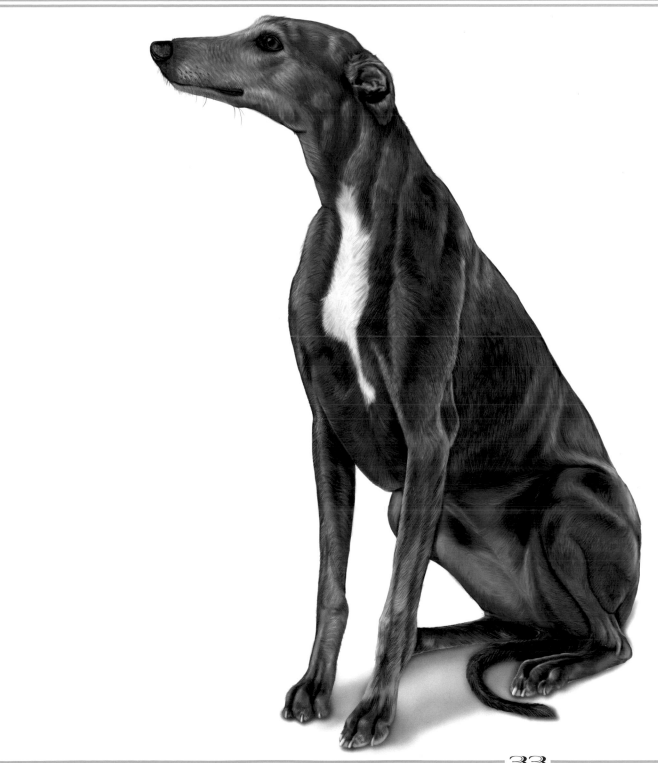

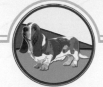

Greyhound

The fastest dog in the world, the Greyhound is also among the most ancient, found in Egyptian drawings from as far back as 2900 B.C. Well known as racetrack dogs, Greyhounds were once used to chase notoriously fast animals like deer and wild boar. Greyhounds have become excellent family pets, as they are good-natured and loyal.

The Greyhound's short, smooth coat can be virtually any color, the most common ones being black, brindle, fawn, and red. Grooming is quick and easy, requiring only an occasional brushing or bath. Greyhounds should sleep in soft, well-cushioned areas, as they are prone to developing pressure sores.

These sweet dogs make excellent playmates for children and dogs familiar to them. Greyhounds chase small animals and should be kept on a leash whenever they are not in a fenced-in area. Greyhounds learn quickly but can become bored easily, making them difficult to train—so an early start is a must. Their masters should be physically fit in order to keep up with the daily exercise the dogs require.

Height . . . . 27–30 in. / 68–76 cm
Weight . . . . 60–70 lb /27–32 kg
Grooming. . . . . low
Exercise. . . . . high
Appetite. . . . . medium
Lifespan. . . . . 8–12 years

Terrier Group

Named after the Latin word for "earth," *terra*, the sprightly dogs known as terriers were bred as far back as the 15th century to dig out and hunt small animals that threatened farms and livestock. Originally developed in the British Isles, terriers were bred more for their vermin-hunting ability than for appearance, so they were not acknowledged as purebreds until almost the 18th century. Now bred as house pets, terriers are energetic, almost tireless dogs that do well with owners of equal enthusiasm. Terriers retain the fighting instinct for which they were originally bred and thus have earned a reputation as willful and somewhat temperamental dogs. While challenging to train, terriers can be among the most engaging and beloved of household pets if handled with a patient firmness from early in life.

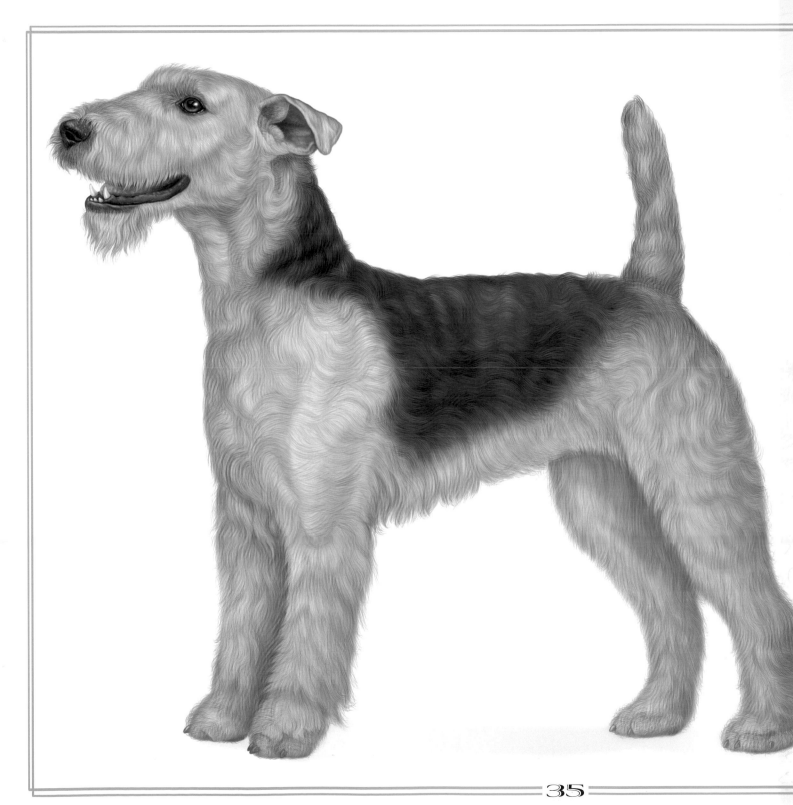

Airedale Terrier

Dubbed the "king of terriers," the Airedale Terrier is the largest of the terrier breeds. A loving dog that also offers protection, this versatile breed was developed in Yorkshire, England, in the 18th century, the result of a Terrier–Otterhound crossbreed. The Airedale had an impressive history as a police dog and wartime messenger until the German Shepherd replaced it in those roles.

The Airedale Terrier is born black and develops a second color, usually tan, as it matures. It commonly develops a saddle of darker fur that covers its back and lower neck. The Airedale's wiry, dense, double coat needs brushing a couple of times a week, plus clipping every one to two months.

As one of the most dependable guard dogs, the Airedale Terrier is also a sweet-natured and gentle playmate for children. Because it may challenge other dogs, it should be supervised around them. Airedales are similar to other terriers in their stubbornness, and obedience training should begin early but should not be too strict. Vigorous, frequent exercise is an absolute requirement.

Height . . . . 22–24 in. / 56–61 cm
Weight . . . . 45–50 lb / 20–23 kg
Grooming . . . . medium
Exercise . . . . high
Appetite . . . . medium
Lifespan . . . . 10–13 years

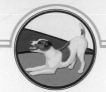

Jack Russell Terrier

Developed to be the ideal hunting dog—small but fearless—the Jack Russell Terrier was extremely popular with hunters in 19th-century England. Reverend John Russell, a famous dog breeder and clergyman, bred the dog to be a fast runner that could also hunt and drive foxes from small ground holes. Lively and energetic, Jack Russells continue to thrive in wide, open spaces today.

The Jack Russell's coat comes in two varieties: smooth or broken. It is normally white, with tan, brown, or black markings around the face, back, and underside. Jack Russells require minimal grooming—an occasional brushing will do.

Obedience training should begin early due to the breed's high energy level and proneness to distraction. Jack Russells should be exposed to children and other animals at an early age if they are to get along well. They will bark when strangers come near their home but otherwise are not aggressive. Ample exercise and room to run are recommended for this dog.

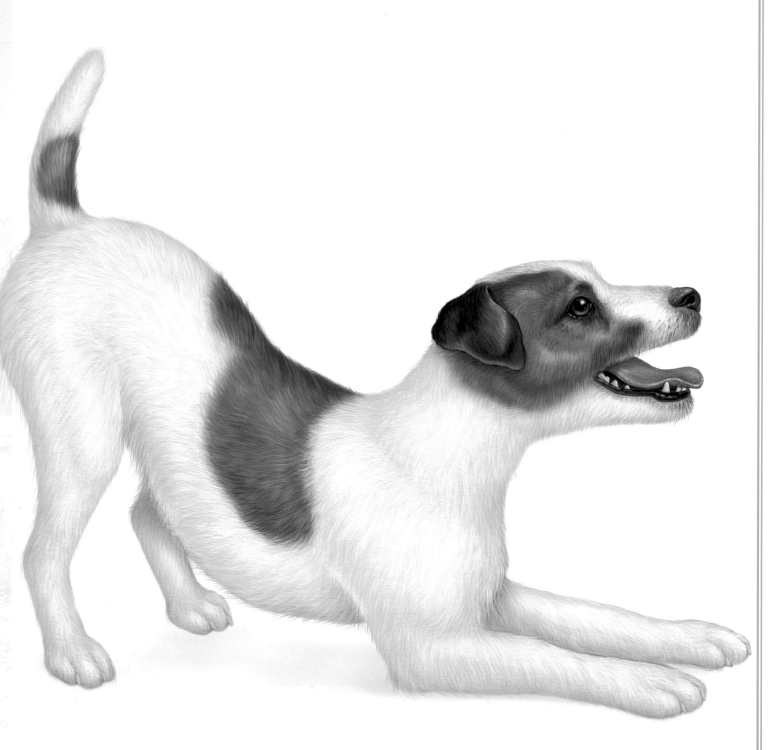

Height . . . . 12–14 in. / 30–35 cm
Weight. . . . . 13–17 lb / 6–8 kg
Grooming. . . . . low
Exercise. . . . . high
Appetite . . . . low
Lifespan . . . . 13–15 years

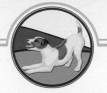

Kerry Blue Terrier

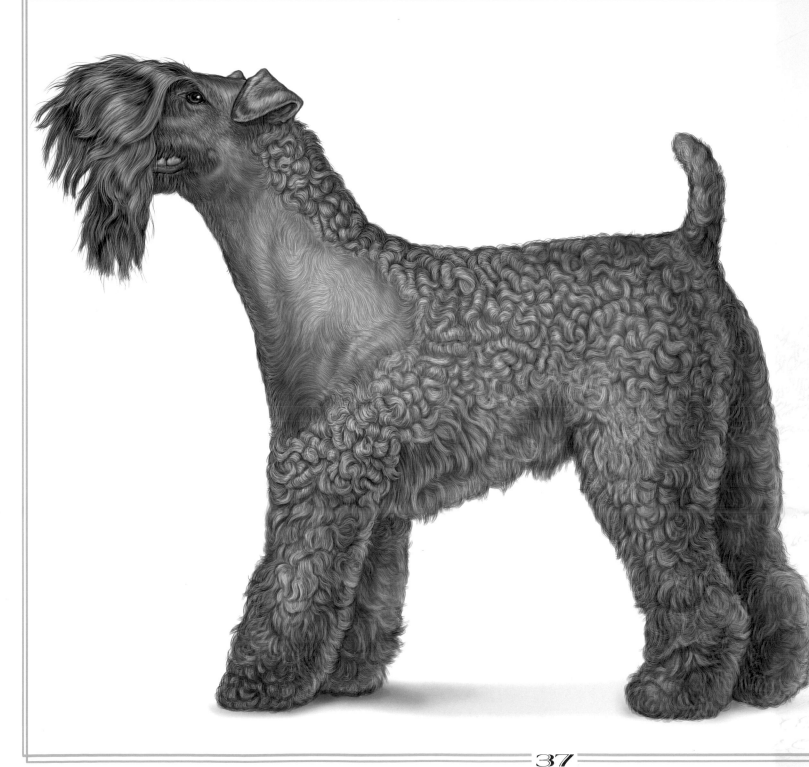

A born watchdog, the Kerry Blue Terrier is commendably loyal and is also admired for its hunting and herding abilities and its distinctive blue-gray coat. The breed originated in the 1700s in Ireland's County Kerry, after which it is named. The Kerry Blue is a true terrier, bred to be a versatile hunter of vermin and small game as well as a retriever and herder.

This graceful, compact dog is born black, but its coat changes to any of a variety of blue, silver, or gray shades between its first and second year of life. Its soft, distinctive coat is completely non-shedding and should be brushed and combed several times a week.

The stubbornness that makes the Kerry Blue Terrier so tenacious in a fight often shows up in obedience training. Owners of Kerry Blues must be patient, yet firm, and training should begin early in life. Ample exercise is essential to keep this breed happy and healthy. Kerry Blues can be aggressive toward other dogs and should be supervised around them.

Height . . . . 17–20 in. / 43–51 cm
Weight . . . . 33–40 lb / 15–18 kg
Grooming . . . . medium
Exercise . . . . high
Appetite . . . . high
Lifespan . . . . 12–15 years

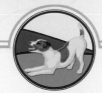

Miniature Schnauzer

Named after the German word *schnauze* (snout), the Miniature Schnauzer is most recognized for the long hair on its muzzle and its distinctive face. This friendly dog was originally bred in Germany to go into the ground and hunt vermin. It is now adored as a family and city-living pet, requiring far less activity than its British terrier counterparts.

The Miniature Schnauzer's face is defined not only by its beard, but also by its bushy eyebrows and high-set, pointy ears. Its coat is wiry and rough and ranges in color from black to salt-and-pepper, which appears gray. Miniature Schnauzers shed minimally and should be combed and brushed once weekly.

As one of the less stubborn and hyperactive of the terrier breeds, Miniature Schnauzers are easy to obedience-train and can skip a day of exercise periodically. They are excellent with children and other animals. Despite their affable nature, Miniature Schnauzers are excellent watchdogs that love to bark—a tendency that should be nipped early if it is excessive.

Height . . . . 12–14 in. /30–35 cm
Weight. . . . . 13–15 lb / 6–7 kg
Grooming. . . . . low
Exercise . . . . medium
Appetite . . . . low
Lifespan . . . . 12–14 years

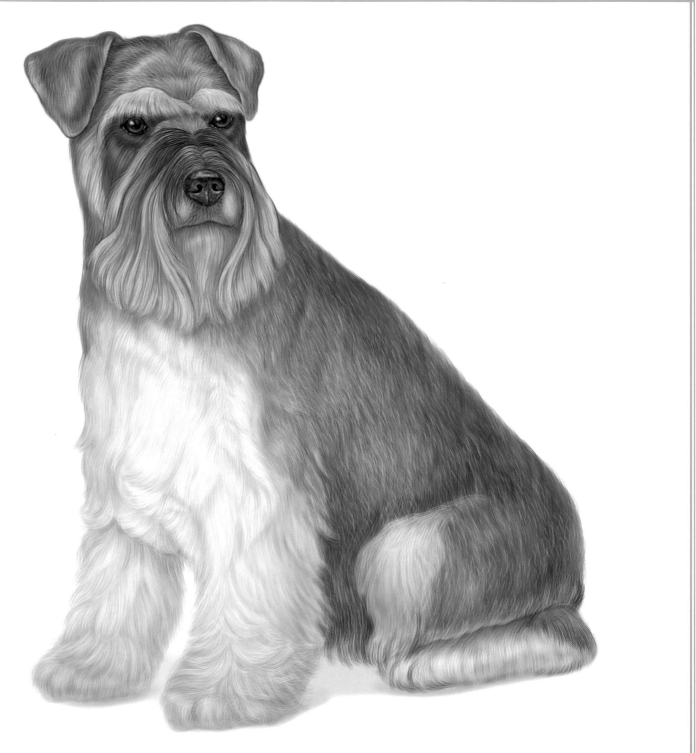

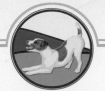

Scottish Terrier

The Scottie, or Scottish Terrier, originated in Aberdeen, Scotland, in the late 1800s to chase small animals such as rabbits and foxes into their dens. The best known Scottie is probably Fala, President Franklin Delano Roosevelt's beloved companion. Indeed, the handsome Scottish Terrier is a proud breed, known for its fierce loyalty to its master—and relative indifference to anyone else.

The Scottish Terrier's characteristic pointy ears become erect around the eighth week of life. Its coat is hard and bristly, with a soft, protective undercoat. Scotties range in color from black to brindle to wheaten and should be brushed a few times a week.

Independent and stubborn, Scotties should be obedience-trained early in life. They are sensitive dogs that require gentle training methods and plenty of praise. Scotties tend to be reserved but friendly with strangers, and they are devoted to their family. They are excellent watchdogs and should be kept on a leash around other animals. Daily walks and playtime are essential.

Height . . . . 10 in. / 25 cm
Weight . . . . 18–22 lb / 8–10 kg
Grooming . . . . medium
Exercise . . . . medium
Appetite . . . . medium
Lifespan . . . . 11–13 years

Working Group

Working dogs are united by the instinct to guard—be it livestock, property, or people. Though other dogs are good guardians, too, none excel as consistently as those in the working group. Bred hundreds of years ago, working dogs are hardy and talented, having been used extensively throughout history as police dogs, wartime dogs, and search and rescue dogs. They are aptly named since they offer outstanding service to those who own them. Unfortunately, the stamina for which working breeds are praised can make them difficult and demanding choices as house pets. Early, intensive obedience training is required for most working dogs if they are to be happy, healthy members of the family. High amounts of vigorous exercise are another general requirement. If given enough training and direction by a strong master, however, working dogs can be very loving and affectionate pets that retain their instinct for duty.

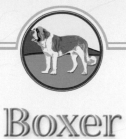

Boxer

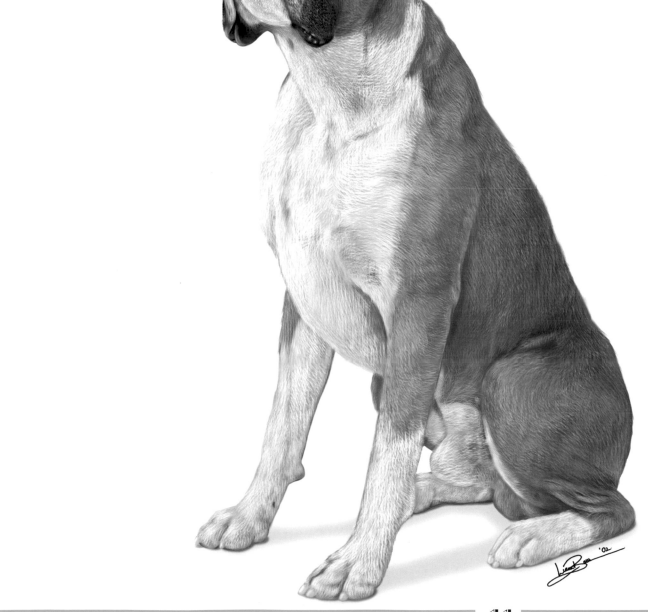

Although the Boxer is something of a perennial child, its fun-loving personality is matched by a capable intelligence that has been put to use by both police and military units throughout history. The Boxer originated in 19th-century Germany as a guard dog and is descended from the now extinct Bullenbeisser. The Boxer is lively in nature and still retains its original guarding instincts.

The Boxer's coat is short, smooth, and shiny. Colors include fawn and brindle, usually with white markings. Boxers can be solid white, though they are disqualified from professional dog shows. Grooming requirements are minimal—occasional brushing and washing will do.

Enthusiastic and playful, Boxers make rewarding companions. Boxers also love children and make the gentlest of playmates for them. They are protective of loved ones and their property and thus make excellent watchdogs. Boxers need thorough obedience training from early on to keep them under control. Although they are not aggressive dogs, they will not back down if other dogs challenge them. Boxers need several walks a day to expend their seemingly endless energy and to avoid becoming overweight.

Height . . . . 21–25 in. / 53–64 cm
Weight . . . . 55–75 lb / 25–34 kg
Grooming . . . . low
Exercise . . . . high
Appetite . . . . medium
Lifespan . . . . 13–15 years

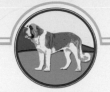

Doberman Pinscher

The fearless, energetic Doberman Pinscher was bred in Germany to be an all-purpose guard dog in the latter half of the 19th century. Smart and unrelenting, the Doberman was used as a wartime dog that bravely participated in combat! Today, Doberman Pinschers are popular as guard dogs. Though not as vicious as some think, Dobermans can be aggressive and need strong masters to keep them under control. With proper training and guidance, Doberman Pinschers can become good family dogs with a capacity for gentleness.

The Doberman Pinscher's coat is short, hard, and smooth. Coat colors include black, red, blue, and fawn, usually with rust-colored markings. This breed sheds little, and grooming with a soft cloth or brush once a week is sufficient.

Though the Doberman was once known for its aggressive nature, this trait has now been curbed due to selective breeding. Still, they are natural protectors, requiring firm and dedicated training. They are very useful and intelligent dogs that obey well. Dobermans require high-speed exercise on a daily basis.

Height . . . . . . 24–28 in. / 61–71 cm
Weight . . . . . . 55–85 lb / 25–39 kg
Grooming . . . . low
Exercise . . . . high
Appetite . . . . high
Lifespan . . . . 10–12 years

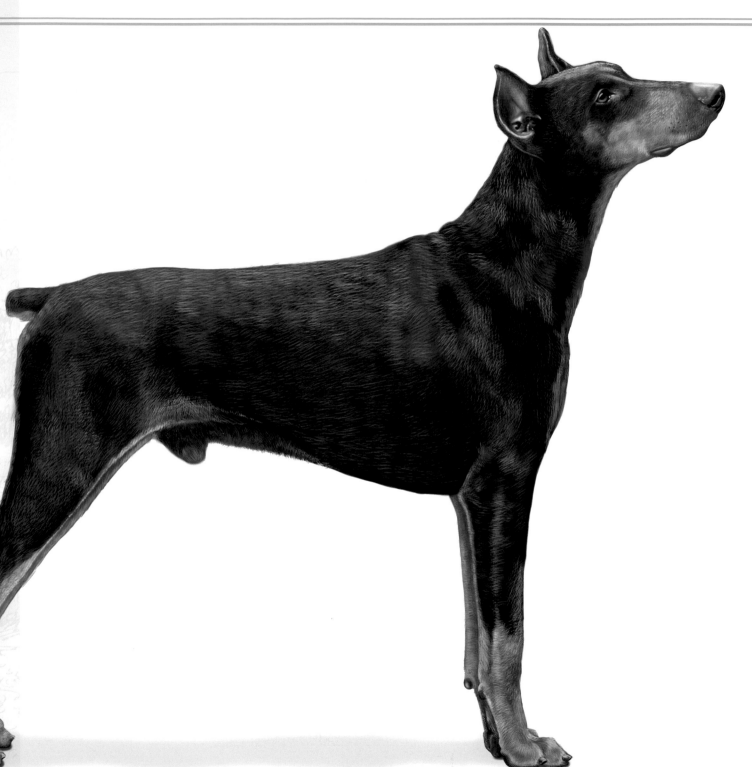

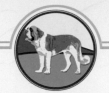

Great Dane

Despite its name, the Great Dane originated in Germany, not in Denmark. Once used to hunt wild boar, the Great Dane is now a loving breed that gets along well with children and other dogs. It offers excellent protection as a watchdog, too, with an imposing appearance to back it up.

The Great Dane's coat is short, smooth, and shiny. Colors include brindle, fawn, steel blue, black, and harlequin, which appears white with broken black spots. Weekly brushing is the only grooming required.

The Great Dane's regal appearance has made it a favorite companion dog, although its personality and skillfulness are equally appealing. Great Danes are spirited and playful with children. They make outstanding watchdogs, yet they are not aggressive with strangers or other dogs. Great Danes are responsive to obedience training, but an early start is important given their large size. Great Danes require less activity than one would suspect; a daily walk is sufficient.

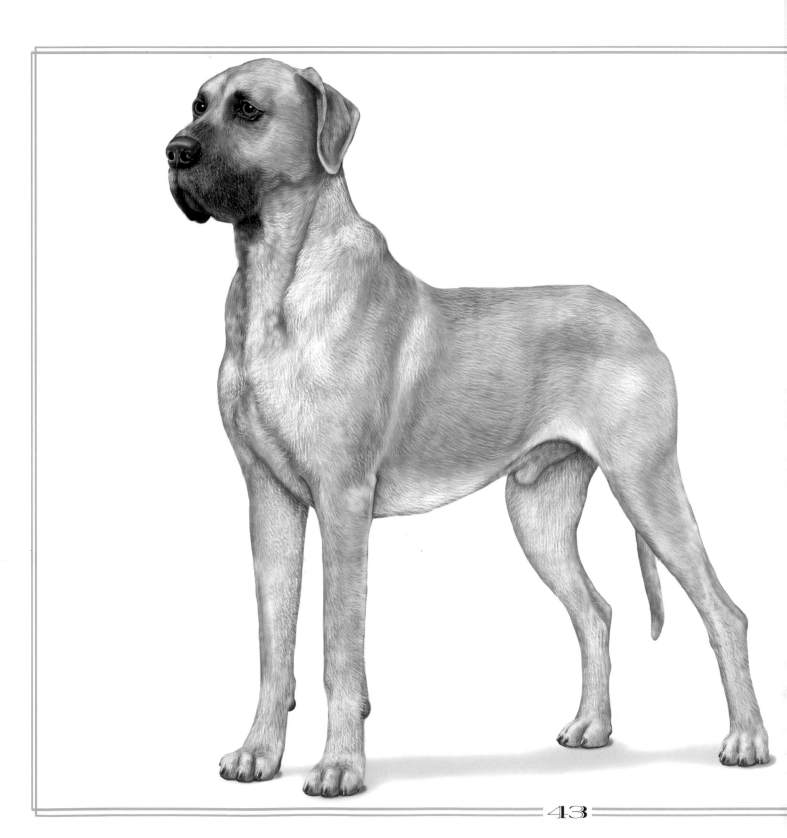

Height	28–32 in. / 71–81 cm
Weight	100–140 lb / 45–63 kg
Grooming	low
Exercise	medium
Appetite	high
Lifespan	9–10 years

Saint Bernard

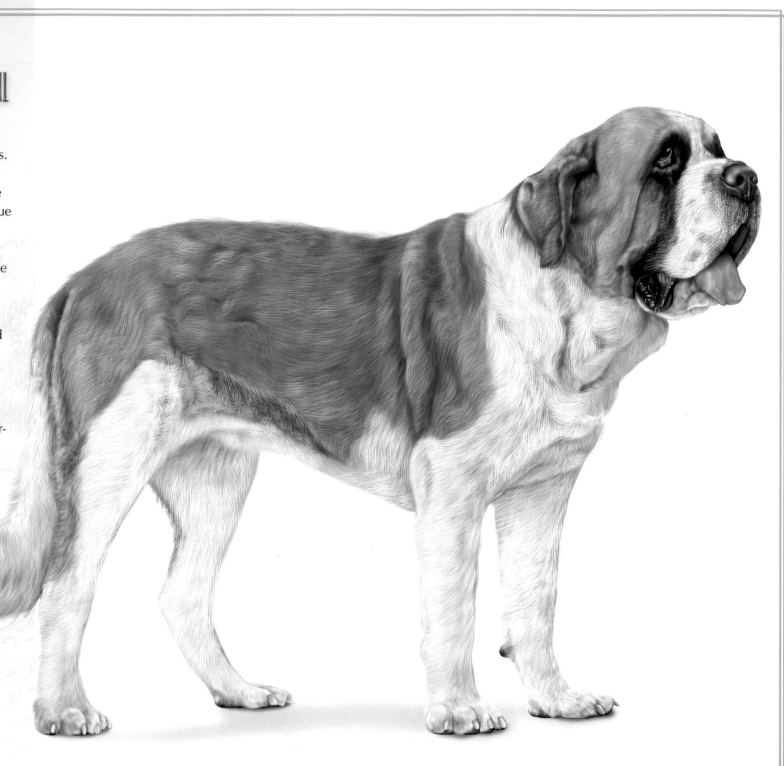

Sweet and oversized, the lovable Saint Bernard originated in Switzerland during the Middle Ages. In the 17th century, Swiss monks adopted the hardy breed as a companionable guard dog. The Saint Bernard was renowned as a search and rescue dog, trailing those lost in the snow and upon finding them, lying down beside them to warm them! Today, the Saint Bernard is a gentle, affable breed that gets along well with almost anybody.

Saint Bernards can be either shorthaired or longhaired. Coat colors are a combination of red and white or of brindle with white markings. Grooming the coat is simple but, frequent brushings are required because Saint Bernards shed continually. Other care includes frequent cleaning of the eyes, which have very active tear-producing glands, and of the ears.

The Saint Bernard is a superb family pet, although its large size must be taken into account. This breed is playful with children and dogs alike, but Saint Bernards still require early obedience training to keep their massive strength under control.

Height . . . . 25–28 in. / 63–71 cm
Weight . . . . 110–200 lb / 50–91 kg
Grooming . . . . medium
Exercise . . . . low
Appetite. high
Lifespan . . . . 8–10 years

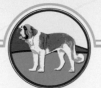

Siberian Husky

The nomadic Chukchi tribe of Siberia bred the Siberian Husky more than three thousand years ago to be a fast and tireless sled dog. The Siberian Husky is the most talented of all the sled dogs and excels in races, due at least in part to its long, friendly relationship with human beings. This breed makes a gentle and energetic house pet.

The Siberian Husky's beautiful and warm coat consists of a smooth, longhaired outercoat and soft, dense undercoat. Coat colors are seen in all combinations. Shedding is rather extensive, making frequent brushing necessary.

Siberian Huskies truly adore people and enjoy spending time with the family, preferably while engaged in some sort of vigorous activity. They need ample exercise and room to run free, but a fenced-in yard is necessary to prevent them from wandering off. These dogs are rarely aggressive and get along well with children and other dogs. Obedience training should begin early, however, because Siberian Huskies can have a mind of their own.

Height . . . . 20–23 in. / 51–59 cm
Weight . . . . 35–60 lb / 16–27 kg
Grooming . . . . high
Exercise . . . . high
Appetite . . . . high
Lifespan . . . . 11–13 years

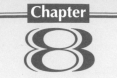
Non-Sporting Group

This diverse group includes the dogs that were not bred for a specific purpose, such as herding, chasing vermin, or hunting. Nevertheless, several members of the non-sporting group are quite good at one or more of these activities and have been used historically for such purposes. These dogs have also enjoyed popularity as circus performers, because they are generally both easy to train and entertaining to watch. Non-sporting breeds are admired today as adaptable companion dogs. The non-sporting dogs are big and small, easygoing and temperamental, and above all, just as lovable as their more purposefully named counterparts.

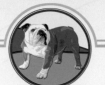

Bichon Frise

The ultimate lap dog, the Bichon Frise was the fair-haired darling of French and Italian aristocratic women during the Renaissance. The exact origins of the Bichon Frise are unclear, although it is thought to date back to the Middle Ages and to be of Mediterranean origin. Playful and born to please, the Bichon Frise is now a favorite family pet.

The Bichon Frise has a luxurious coat consisting of two layers: a soft, silky undercoat and a coarse, curly outercoat. Its color is an opulent white, often with shades of buff, apricot, or cream. The naturally curly coat is usually groomed to be fluffy, much like a poodle, but this requires brushing for at least one-half hour a day and monthly trimming. If left natural, the coat still requires frequent brushing.

This breed is adored for its lively and endearing personality and for its friendly spirit with children and other pets. The Bichon Frise loves to earn praise, making obedience training fun and easy. Minimal exercise is needed beyond daily playtime.

Height	9–11 in. / 24–29 cm
Weight	7–12 lb / 3–5 kg
Grooming	medium–high
Exercise	low
Appetite	low
Lifespan	12–15 years

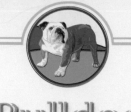

Bulldog

The now-friendly Bulldog once used its characteristic muzzle to bait bulls by latching onto their noses. When bull baiting was banned in England in 1835, the ferocious Bulldog was transformed through selective breeding into an amiable and mellow house pet. Instead of chasing bulls, the Bulldog is now most content to spend its days playing with children and lolling around the house.

Because of their large heads, Bulldogs usually must be born via Cesarean section. Their color at birth remains the same throughout their lives, and their coats consist of brindle, white, red, or fawn. The hair is short and soft and requires a quick brushing once a week. The area between the folds around the muzzle should be cleaned more regularly.

Like a big teddy bear, the Bulldog is good with children and makes an excellent playmate. Bulldogs enjoy the company of dogs that they have been raised with, although some can be aggressive with unfamiliar dogs. Generally reserved and good-natured, the Bulldog can be stubborn but is generally not difficult to train. It needs minimal exercise and, in fact, should avoid prolonged exertion.

Height . . . . 12–15 in. / 30–38 cm
Weight. . . . . 40–50 lb / 18–23 kg
Grooming. . . . . low
Exercise . . . . low
Appetite. . . . . medium
Lifespan . . . . 8–10 years

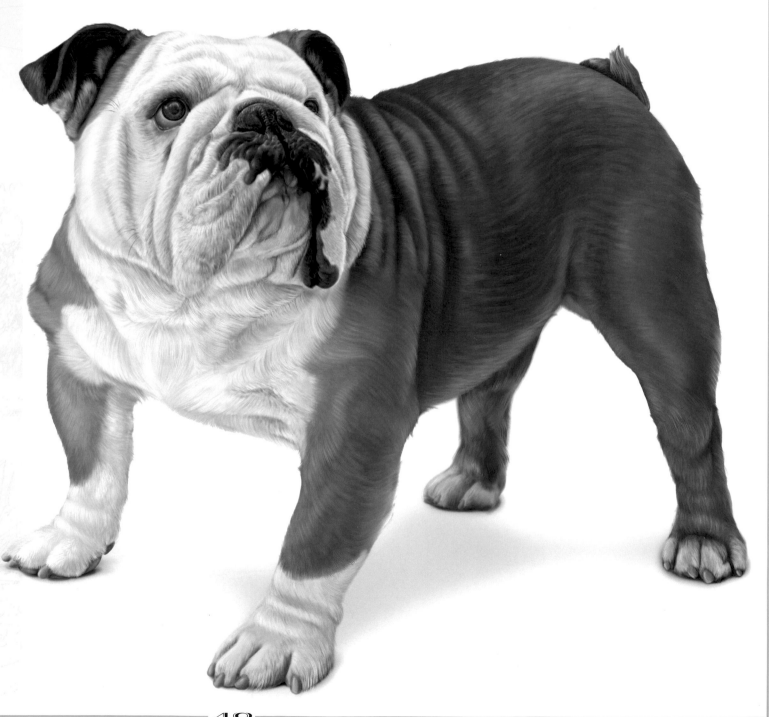

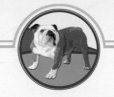

Chow Chow

With its lion-like looks and unique, stilted gait, the two-thousand-year-old Chow Chow was admired in ancient China for both its beauty and its skill. Developed to hunt and herd, the Chow Chow was prized for its stunning fur and was even eaten as a delicacy! Today, the Chow Chow remains regal in appearance but is most suited to have one devoted master.

The Chow Chow's coat can be smooth or rough, and its color can be cream, fawn, red, blue, or black. The plush coat consists of straight hair on top and an undercoat that is woolly and dense. Grooming requirements are extensive and include daily combing of the undercoat and brushing of the outercoat. Chow Chows shed quite a bit, too.

Though devoted to their masters, Chow Chows can be aloof and suspicious of strangers. Chow Chows can be aggressive toward other dogs but are usually good with other household pets. Early obedience training and socialization are essential, as this can be a challenging breed to teach. Chow Chows make excellent watchdogs and require little exercise.

Height	17–20 in./ 43–51cm
Weight	45–70 lb / 20–32 kg
Grooming	high
Exercise	low
Appetite	medium
Lifespan	8–12 years

Dalmatian

The Dalmatian is thought to have originated in the region of Dalmatia, now part of Croatia. Artistic renderings of the Dalmatian have been found on ancient Egyptian and Greek friezes. Eighteenth-century British aristocrats adored this all-purpose dog that guarded them, their carriages, and their horses. The Dalmatian is an energetic and intelligent dog that continues to serve as a circus performer and as a firehouse mascot.

The unique and most recognizable feature of the Dalmatian is its vividly spotted coat, which is pure white at birth; black or liver spots develop as the dog matures. Dalmatians require a weekly brushing to prevent excessive shedding. The smart, vivacious Dalmatian is quite clean and even enjoys baths!

Dalmatians crave contact with those they love and can play for hours with children, though they should be supervised around young children as Dalmations may be too energetic for them. Because they can be aloof toward strangers as well as stubborn, socialization and obedience training should begin early. Dalmatians need plenty of aerobic exercise to remain well behaved.

Height . . . . 19-24 in. / 48–61 cm
Weight . . . . 45–60 lb / 20–27 kg
Grooming . . . . medium
Exercise . . . . high
Appetite . . . . low
Lifespan . . . . 12–14 years

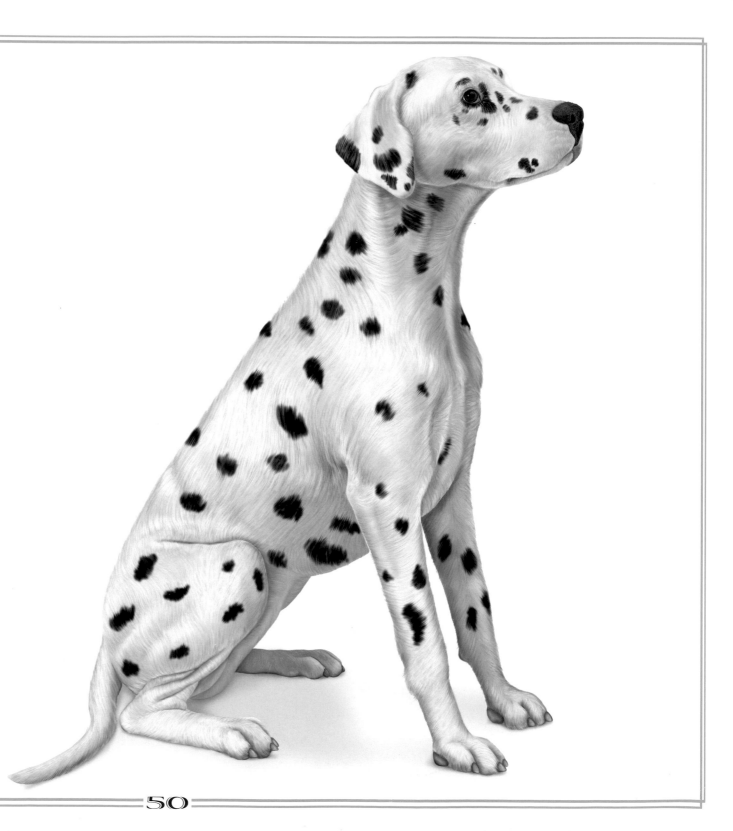

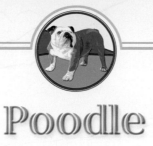

Poodle

Considered the national dog of France, the Poodle originated in Germany as far back as the Middle Ages. Taking its name from the German word *pudeln*, which means "to splash in water," the Poodle was once exceptional at retrieving ducks from marshes. The versatile Poodle is among the most intelligent and capable of breeds. It is easily trained and thus remains a popular family pet to this day.

The Poodle has a beautiful coat that is single-layer and completely non-shedding. Poodles are always unicolored and can be black, white, apricot, brown, cream, silver, or blue. They require brushing a few times a week, plus clipping and shaping every four to six weeks.

The responsive, full-of-personality Poodle is a talented dog in all social arenas. It loves children, gets along well with other animals, and is easy to obedience-train. One thing Poodles do require is plenty of exercise. While there are three types of Poodles, the Standard, Miniature, and Toy—only the Standard and Miniature belong to the non-sporting group.

Height	Standard	>15 in. / >38 cm
	Miniature	10–15 in. / 13–23 cm
Weight	Standard	45–70 lb / 20–32 kg
	Miniature	26–30 lb / 12–14 kg
Grooming		medium–high
Exercise		high
Appetite		medium
Lifespan		10–13 years

Toy Group

The toy group could be referred to as the companion dog group, because this is its member breeds' foremost purpose. Toy dogs, in many cases, have been providing love and companionship for several thousand years. They excel at creating warm, affectionate bonds with their masters and are devoted pets in general. This group of dogs, more than any other, especially craves human contact and requires attentive owners. Not simply ornaments, toy dogs are vivacious. Many make excellent watchdogs and can hold their own with dogs much larger than themselves. Toy dogs are ideal for city living; in addition, they are much less expensive to maintain, and cleaning up after them is easier than with larger breeds. The toy group is a diverse collection of diminutive dogs that assimilate well into households everywhere. All dogs in this group, however, should be watched closely when they are around children, as their small size can make them vulnerable to injury from roughhousing.

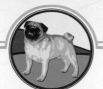

Chihuahua

As the smallest of all breeds, the Chihuahua has ancient origins that are not entirely clear. It is said to have been descended from the Techicchi, a sacred dog among the Toltec and Aztec tribes of the ninth century. Remains of the Chihuahua have been found in ancient human graves in both Mexico and the United States. Like many of the toy breeds, the Chihuahua has a big, bold personality despite its tiny size. Alert and dominant, Chihuahuas form strong attachments to their masters and seek to protect them by acting as watchdogs.

Chihuahuas come in two varieties: smooth and longhaired. Coats can be nearly any color, and an occasional brushing is the only grooming required for both varieties.

The Chihuahua is gentle and playful with children, but it needs supervision to avoid injury from roughhousing. Aside from their size, Chihuahuas are hardy dogs that love activity and exercise. They are easy to train and adore their masters. Chihuahuas can be friendly with other dogs, but they prefer the company of other Chihuahuas instead!

Height . . . . 6–9 in. / 15–23 cm
Weight. . . . . 2–6 lb / 1–3 kg
Grooming. . . . . low
Exercise . . . . low
Appetite . . . . low
Lifespan . . . . 13–15 years

L. Kwong

Japanese Chin

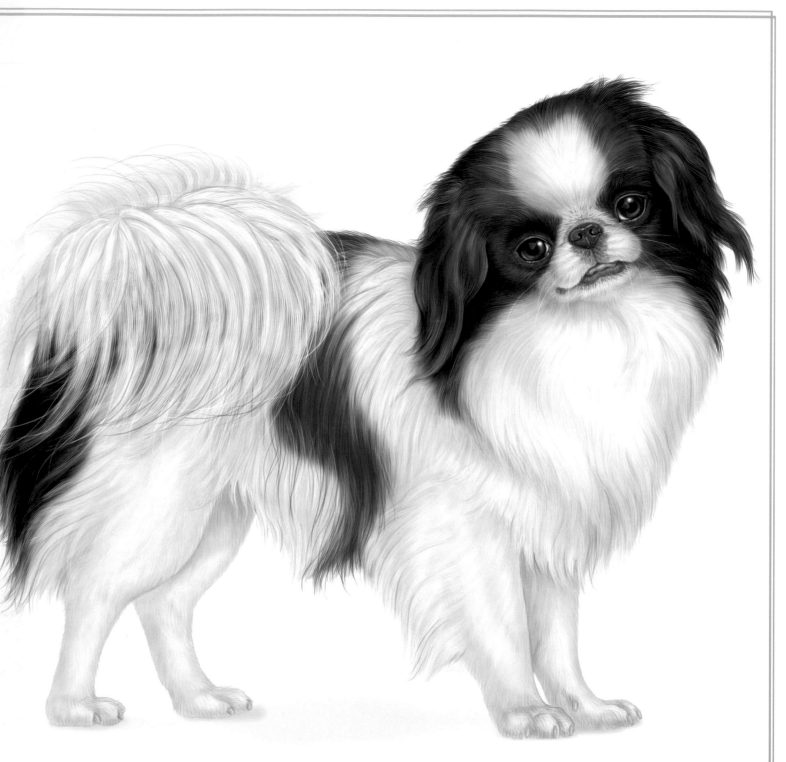

Presumably originating in China, the Japanese Chin was brought to Japan about A.D. 700 and became a favorite of royalty there. The Japanese Chin was originally known as the Japanese Spaniel, until it became clear that the breed had no relation to the spaniel and it was given its current name. In Japanese, *chin* means "royalty," and the Japanese Chin's name reflects this breed's one-time popularity as a lap dog of the powerful and wealthy. Today, the Japanese Chin remains a gentle companion dog that enjoys people and other animals.

The Japanese Chin's abundant, silky coat is long, with a feathering mane around the neck. Coat color is a combination either of black and white or of red and white. Despite its luxurious look, the coat is simple to groom and requires a quick brushing twice a week.

Devoted and affectionate, the Japanese Chin is simple to obedience-train and enjoys the company of people. This breed is playful with children, but it does not tolerate rough handling and should be supervised around the young. Japanese Chins require very little exercise and live happily even in the smallest living areas.

Height . . . . 8–10 in. / 20–25 cm
Weight. . . . . 4–7 lb / 2–3 kg
Grooming. . . . . low
Exercise . . . . low
Appetite . . . . low
Lifespan . . . . 12–14 years

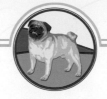

Pug

Once a companion to Tibetan monks, the ancient Pug was miniaturized from the Mastiff more than two thousand years ago. Holland's king and aristocracy later came to love this striking-looking dog. It is no wonder the Pug has enjoyed such tremendous regard throughout history—it is a loving and enthusiastic dog that treats its human family with good-natured loyalty and a fun-loving spirit.

The Pug's short, glossy coat is soft to the touch and easy to groom—one quick brushing a week will do. Coat colors include fawn, apricot, silver, and black. A dark mask around the muzzle and eyes is common.

Pugs are distinctive in that they have a tendency to grunt like pigs in order to communicate with people! This endearing dog also snores when it sleeps. Pugs are intelligent and learn easily, although they can be defiant at times. They are rarely aggressive, and they play well with children and other animals. Pugs require moderate exercise and should not be permitted to become finicky eaters. Pugs cannot tolerate hot weather, indoors or out.

Height . . . . 10–11 in. / 25–28 cm
Weight. . . . . 14–18 lb / 6–8 kg
Grooming. . . . . low
Exercise . . . . medium
Appetite. . . . . medium
Lifespan . . . . 12–15 years

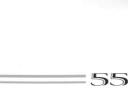

Shih Tzu

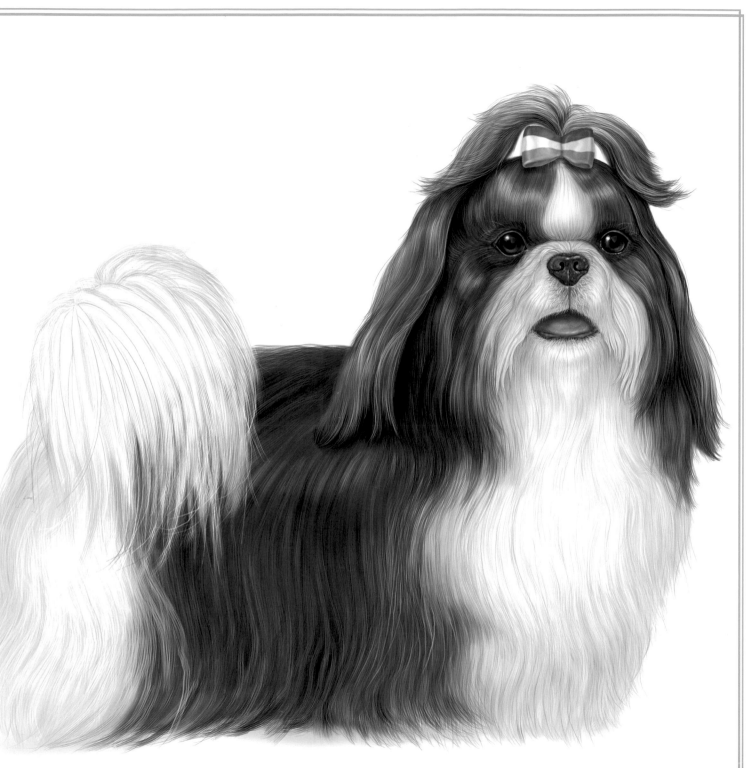

The Shih Tzu takes its name from the Chinese word for "lion" because of its long, lion-like coat. The breed is believed to have origins in ancient China; carvings and paintings of the Shih Tzu have been found from as far back as the seventh century. Another favorite of the royal and aristocratic, the Shih Tzu is a lovable dog that adores children and often lives to 14 years of age!

The Shih Tzu's lavish coat, which can be almost any color, is long on top and dense underneath. Grooming requirements are extensive because the coat can easily become dingy-looking if neglected. Daily combing and brushing are needed. This breed typically needs to have the hair around its face pulled up in a clip to prevent eye irritation and infection.

The affectionate Shih Tzu is a true companion dog that thrives when it is part of the family. This breed loves children, but as with all dogs in the toy group, it should be supervised to avoid mishaps. Shih Tzus are easy to obedience-train, although quick lessons are best because their attention span can be short. They require little exercise.

Height . . . . 8–11 in. / 20–28 cm
Weight. . . . . 9–16 lb / 4–7 kg
Grooming . . . . high
Exercise . . . . low
Appetite . . . . low
Lifespan . . . . 12–14 years

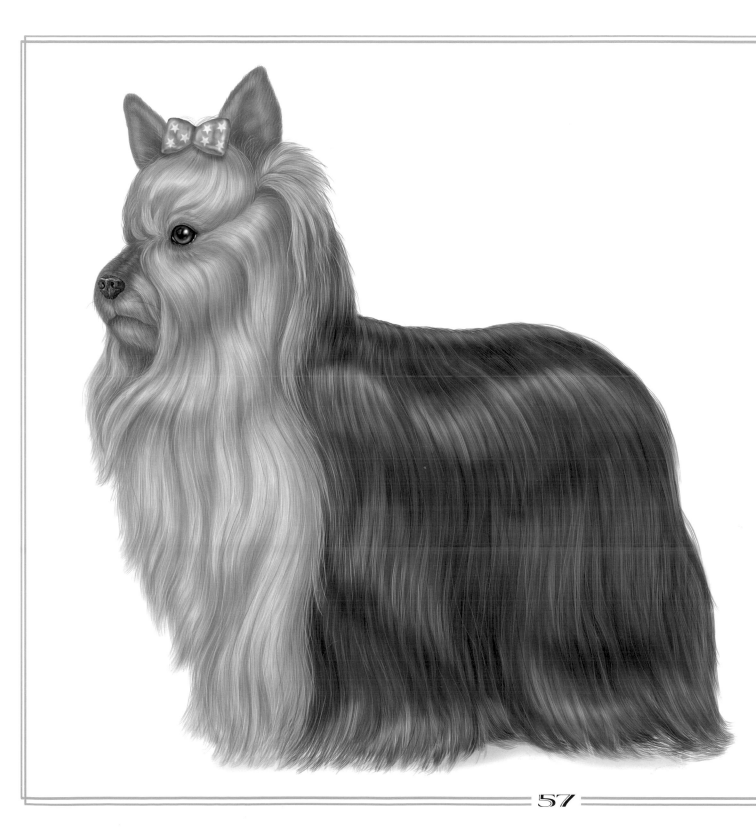

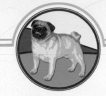

Yorkshire Terrier

Dominant and spirited, the Yorkshire Terrier likes to rule. This pint-sized breed stands up to the largest of dogs and often emerges as the winner in a battle of wills. The Yorkie was developed about one hundred years ago by English miners for the purpose of catching rats. A true terrier, the Yorkie is energetic, loyal to its master, and suspicious of strangers. Today, it is one of the most popular toy breeds worldwide.

The Yorkie's long, glossy coat goes all the way to the ground and requires daily combing and brushing. The hair on its head is usually tied up or parted in the middle. Coat color is always steel blue on the body and golden around the face.

Yorkies have almost unlimited energy and enjoy many types of activities. They like children and belie their size with the vigor and courage they show when playing. This breed is quite small, though, and should be supervised to avoid injury. Yorkies can be stubborn but can be relatively easy to obedience-train. They need little outside exercise and do not tolerate being left alone for long intervals.

Height . . . . 7–8 in. / 18–20 cm
Weight. . . . . 3–7 lb / 1–3 kg
Grooming . . . . high
Exercise . . . . low
Appetite . . . . low
Lifespan . . . . 13–15 years

Herding Group

The function of this group of dogs is obvious, yet remarkable: To herd and direct animals, often much larger than themselves, to pasture or other destinations. Shepherds bred herding dogs hundreds of years ago to help maintain and control their livestock. Most dogs in this group were developed to herd either cattle or sheep by nipping at their heels and charging or leaping in front of them. Active and intelligent, these dogs were admired both for their trainability and for the service they provided to their owners. Today, herding dogs are admired as lively family pets. Though most will never find a herd of cattle or sheep to chase, they retain their instinct to work and need ample activity and space to remain at their best.

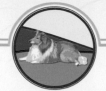

Australian Shepherd

The origins of the Australian Shepherd are murky. It is said to have appeared in the 1800s in California, bred to work as a herding and guard dog for the unique desert-like climate there. Though brought to North America by way of Australia, for which it is named, the breed probably originated in the Basque region of the Pyrenees, a mountain range along the Spanish-French border. Whatever its history, the Australian Shepherd is an excellent working dog that has now adapted to life as a popular family pet.

This breed's generous coat is long and coarse on top, with a soft, dense undercoat. Coat colors include blue merle, red merle, black, and red, sometimes with white and/or tan markings. Grooming is easy and involves only a weekly brushing.

Australian Shepherds love children and get along well with most people. They are trusting animals that seek out interaction with people and other animals. Obedience training is generally simple and enjoyable. They require daily exercise.

Height . . . . 18–23 in. / 46–58 cm
Weight . . . . 35–70 lb / 16–32 kg
Grooming . . . . low
Exercise . . . . high
Appetite . . . . medium
Lifespan . . . . 12–14 years

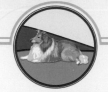

Bouvier des Flandres

A physically powerful and talented breed, the Bouvier des Flandres originated in the 17th century in a region between Belgium and France. Bred to herd cattle and pull milk carts, the Bouvier des Flandres nearly disappeared after World War I due to the violent fighting in its native region. Fortunately, the breed was revived; now the Bouvier, known for its intelligence and physical prowess, is often used as a guard dog or military dog. The Bouvier des Flandres is a true outdoor dog that does not tolerate being cooped up and left inside.

The Bouvier des Flandres' harsh outercoat and dense undercoat enable it to withstand the roughest weather conditions. Its coat, which may be fawn, black, gray, or brindle, requires brushing several times a week to prevent matting.

Because the Bouvier likes to dominate, early socialization and obedience training are important. The Bouvier des Flandres is an excellent watchdog—wary of strangers and protective of children and property. Abundant exercise and room to run are essential for this breed's well-being.

Height . . . . 23–27 in. / 60–70 cm
Weight . . . . 65–90 lb / 29–41 kg
Grooming . . . . high
Exercise . . . . high
Appetite . . . . medium
Lifespan . . . . 12–15 years

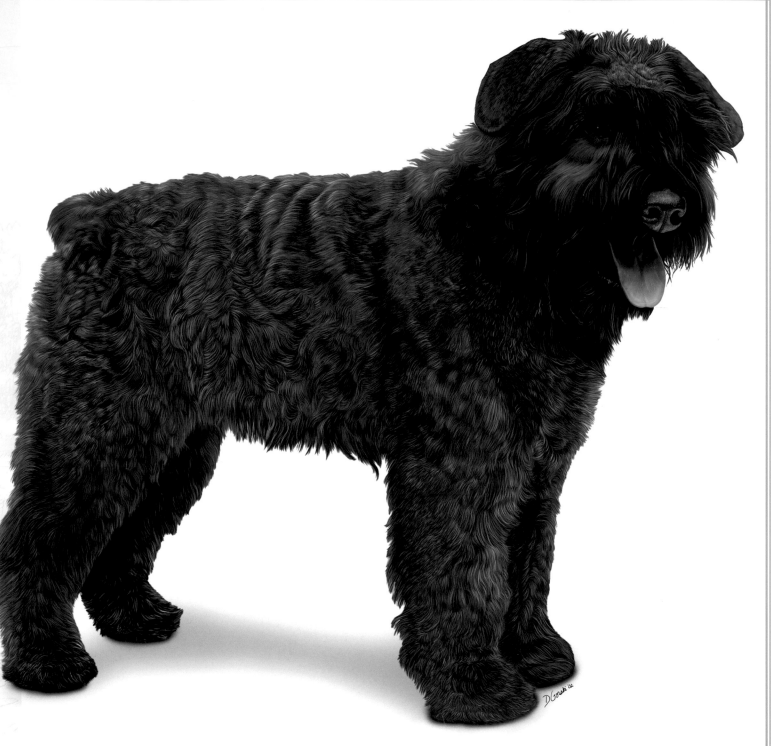

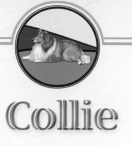

Collie

The Collie lives up to film and television hero Lassie's reputation as a delightful and stunning dog. Originally bred as a cattle- and sheep-herding dog in 19th-century Scotland, the Collie also has been used as a rescue and guard dog due to its high intelligence. Today, Collies make loving and gentle pets that are among the most beautiful and popular of all breeds.

The Collie's coat comes in two varieties: rough and smooth. The rough coat consists of a straight and abundant outercoat and a soft, dense undercoat, and its fur feathers around the neck. The smooth coat is short, hard, and flat with a nice texture. Both varieties can be sable and white, tricolor, blue merle, or all white. Collies require daily brushing to prevent matting.

Collies adore children and love to spend time with their owners. They are eager to learn, making obedience training easy and fast. The Collie's good nature means it is not aggressive with other dogs or people. This breed can be protective of its family but tends to become friendly with strangers rather easily. Collies require moderate exercise.

Height . . . . 22–26 in. / 56–66 cm
Weight . . . . 50–75 lb / 23–34 kg
Grooming . . . . high
Exercise . . . . medium
Appetite . . . . medium
Lifespan . . . . 11–13 years

German Shepherd Dog

The German Shepherd originated in 19th-century Germany as a sheep-herding dog. Following World War I, it earned widespread acclaim in England because of its excellent wartime performance as a messenger and ambulance dog. Due to anti-German sentiment at the time, it was referred to as the Alsatian and only regained its original name in 1971. Among the most intelligent and agile of dogs, the German Shepherd has become the most popular breed worldwide and is versatile as a police dog, guide dog and a companion dog.

The German Shepherd's coat is straight and harsh on top, with a dense, woolly undercoat. Its color is usually black, tan, gray, or white, although white is disqualified from AKC competition. Frequent brushing is recommended, as German Shepherds shed constantly.

These talented dogs enjoy being put to use and can behave problematically if not given daily attention. Intelligent and easy to train, German Shepherds are protective of loved ones and property. They are wary of strangers and make excellent watchdogs. Plenty of exercise is essential.

Height . . . . 22–26 in. / 56–66 cm
Weight . . . . 60–100 lb / 27–45 kg
Grooming . . . . medium
Exercise . . . . high
Appetite . . . . medium
Lifespan . . . . 11–13 years

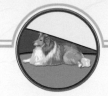

Welsh Corgi (Pembroke)

The smallest member of the herding group, the Welsh Corgi takes its name from the Welsh for "dwarf dog." Flemish weavers brought the Pembroke Welsh Corgi, one of two Corgi breeds, to Wales in the 11th century. Small but capable, the Pembroke was bred to herd cattle, moving the cows along by nipping at their heels and ankles with amazing success. These capable and spirited dogs now make excellent family pets, although they sometimes try to "herd" people by nipping at their heels! The Pembroke is a first-rate companion dog that still likes to work.

The Pembroke's outer coat is straight and coarse, the undercoat short and dense. Coat colors include red, sable, fawn, or black and tan, sometimes with white markings. Brushing once a week is adequate.

Friendly, energetic, and smart, the Pembroke is an enjoyable pet to have around. Pembrokes are easy to obedience-train, and they are good with children and other dogs. They can be wary of strangers initially and make good watchdogs for this reason. Daily exercise will keep the Pembroke's weight under control.

Height . . . . 10–12 in. / 25–30 cm
Weight . . . . 20–30 lb / 9–13 kg
Grooming . . . . low
Exercise . . . . medium
Appetite . . . . medium
Lifespan . . . . 11–13 years

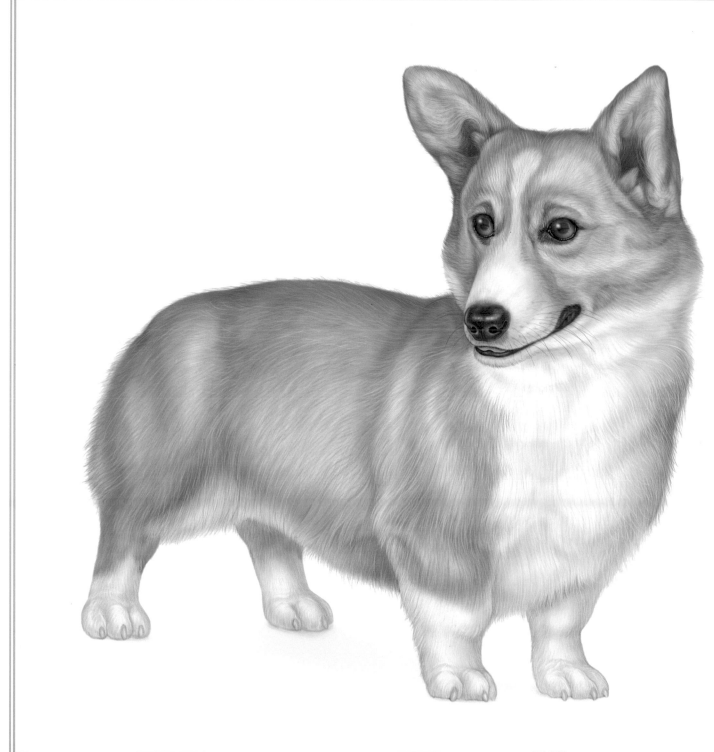

American Kennel Club Recognized Breeds

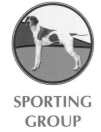

SPORTING GROUP

Brittany
Pointer
German Shorthaired Pointer
German Wirehaired Pointer
Chesapeake Bay Retriever
Curly-Coated Retriever
Flat-Coated Retriever
Golden Retriever
Labrador Retriever
English Setter
Gordon Setter
Irish Setter
American Water Spaniel
Clumber Spaniel
Cocker Spaniel
English Cocker Spaniel
English Springer Spaniel
Field Spaniel
Irish Water Spaniel
Spinone Italiano
Sussex Spaniel
Welsh Springer Spaniel
Vizsla
Weimaraner
Wirehaired Pointing Griffon

HOUND GROUP

Afghan Hound
Basenji
Basset Hound
Beagle
Black and Tan Coonhound
Bloodhound
Borzoi
Dachshund
Foxhound (American)
Foxhound (English)
Greyhound
Harrier
Ibizan Hound
Irish Wolfhound
Norwegian Elkhound
Otterhound
Petit Basset Griffon Vendeen
Pharaoh Hound
Rhodesian Ridgeback
Saluki
Scottish Deerhound
Whippet

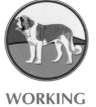

WORKING GROUP

Akita
Alaskan Malamute
Anatolian Shepherd
Bernese Mountain Dog
Boxer
Bullmastiff
Doberman Pinscher
Giant Schnauzer
Great Dane
Great Pyrenees
Greater Swiss Mountain Dog
Komondor
Kuvasz
Mastiff
Newfoundland
Portuguese Water Dog
Rottweiler
Saint Bernard
Samoyed
Siberian Husky
Standard Schnauzer

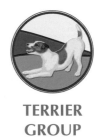

TERRIER GROUP

Airedale Terrier
American Staffordshire Terrier
Australian Terrier
Bedlington Terrier
Border Terrier
Bull Terrier
Cairn Terrier
Dandie Dinmont Terrier
Fox Terrier (Smooth)
Fox Terrier (Wire)
Irish Terrier
Jack Russell Terrier
Kerry Blue Terrier
Lakeland Terrier
Manchester Terrier (Standard)
Miniature Bull Terrier
Miniature Schnauzer
Norfolk Terrier
Norwich Terrier
Scottish Terrier
Sealyham Terrier
Skye Terrier
Soft Coated Wheaten Terrier
Staffordshire Bull Terrier
Welsh Terrier
West Highland White Terrier

TOY GROUP

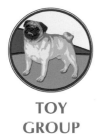

Affenpinscher
Brussels Griffon
Cavalier King Charles Spaniel
Chihuahua
Chinese Crested
English Toy Spaniel
Havanese
Italian Greyhound
Japanese Chin
Maltese
Manchester Terrier
Miniature Pinscher
Papillon
Pekingese
Pomeranian
Poodle
Pug
Shih Tzu
Silky Terrier
Yorkshire Terrier

NON-SPORTING GROUP

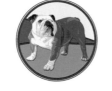

American Eskimo Dog
Bichon Frise
Boston Terrier
Bulldog
Chinese Shar-pei
Chow Chow
Dalmatian
Finnish Spitz
French Bulldog
Keeshond
Lhasa Apso
Löwchen
Poodle
Schipperke
Shiba Inu
Tibetan Spaniel
Tibetan Terrier

HERDING GROUP

Australian Cattle Dog
Australian Shepherd
Bearded Collie
Belgian Malinois
Belgian Sheepdog
Belgian Tervuren
Border Collie
Bouvier des Flandres
Briard
Canaan Dog
Collie
German Shepherd Dog
Old English Sheepdog
Polish Lowland Sheepdog
Puli
Shetland Sheepdog
Welsh Corgi (Cardigan)
Welsh Corgi (Pembroke)

MISCELLANEOUS

Beauceron
Black Russian Terrier
German Pinscher
Glen of Imaal Terrier
Neapolitan Mastiff
Nova Scotia Duck Tolling Retriever
Plott Hound
Redbone Coonhound
Toy Fox Terrier

Credits

❧ Urszula Adamowska, B.F.A.
Like all living animals Urszula requires a balanced diet to grow normally and maintain health once when she matures (this is never going to happen). Urszula grew up in Poland but earned her B.F.A. in Graphic Design at Columbia College, Chicago, her home for the last 12 years. During this time she was trying to 'keep up with the Jones', until coming to the Anatomical Chart Company. She is independent and honest, but having fun with her friends and family is where you'll probably find her! When asked which type of dog she would want to be, Urszula answered, "I would be an Otterhound, because it has a cheerful disposition and enjoys human companionship." Otterhounds can, however, be stubbornly independent—just like Urszula.

❧ Liana Bauman, M.A.M.S.
A native of Arlington Heights, Illinois, Liana received her master of associated medical sciences degree from the University of Illinois at Chicago in 1998. After graduation she was employed by Biomedia Corporation as a medical-legal illustrator. Liana is currently employed as a full-time medical illustrator by the Anatomical Chart Company in Skokie, Illinois. Liana has been a member of the Association of Medical Illustrators (AMI) since 1999 and has received two Certificates of Merit from the AMI for her artwork. "Which Type of Dog would Liana Be?" Friends say—an Australian Terrier, because she is a friendly extrovert with an alert expression and since Australian Terriers are only 10 inches tall, she wouldn't cost a lot to feed.

❧ Dana Demas
Dana grew up in Lake Bluff, Illinois and graduated from the University of Vermont with a bachelor's degree in English and psychology. After college, Dana worked in public relations and then moved to New York City, where she worked in daytime television for two years. Now back in Chicago, she hopes to continue her work as a freelance writer, and someday to publish her own work. Which type of Dog Would She Be? A Beagle, because they are adorable and curious, and perennially childlike.

❧ Dawn Gorski, M.A.M.S.
Dawn received her master's in biomedical illustration from the University of Illinois at Chicago in 1998. Following graduation, she worked at Blausen Medical Communications in Houston, Texas. Missing the great city of Chicago as well as family and friends, she headed back to her hometown and is now working at the Anatomical Chart Company in Skokie, Illinois. Dawn and her pet fish, Fische, enjoy trips to the local aquarium to try to find his real mother. Which Type of Dog would Dawn Be? A Bernese Mountain Dog, because it is a cheerful, intelligent pet and a wonderful companion.

❧ M.S.A. Kumar, D.V.M., Ph.D.
Dr. Kumar obtained his veterinary degree from Mysore Veterinary College in India. He has also received master's degrees in anatomy and physiology as well as a Ph.D. in neuroscience from the University of Florida. For the last 25 years he has taught veterinary gross anatomy, histology, and embryology to veterinary students in India, Nigeria, and Florida. Currently, he is the director of veterinary anatomy programs at Tufts University in North Grafton, Massacheussets. Dr. Kumar has published approximately one hundred scientific papers, abstracts, and book chapters on various topics in neuroscience. His current research is on the effects of nitrous oxide and lead on the neuroendocrine system. Dr. Kumar says he would like to be a Collie because, they bond well with people, and they lead easy going, outdoor lives.

❧ Lik Kwong, M.F.A.
Lik earned his B.F.A. in graphic design and his M.F.A. in medical illustration from the University of Michigan. After graduation, he worked at the university's Department of Biocommunication and then at Allison Legal Graphics in Miami, Florida. Now a Chicago resident, he works at the Anatomical Chart Company as a senior medical illustrator producing new charts and products for educational and pharmaceutical clients. As a member of the Association of Medical Illustrators, he received an Award of Excellence in Instructional Color for his "Understanding Human DNA"chart. Lik would be a Manchester Terrier, because they are handsome, active, and affectionate companions.

❧ Nancy Liskar
A native of the Chicago area, Nancy is a Phi Beta Kappa graduate of Washington University in St. Louis. in her twenty-plus years as a professional editor, she has enjoyed a long association with the Anatomical Chart Company and has edited magazines, journals, newsletters, catalogs, books, and other print communications for several other organizations. Although she would like to own a dog someday, she doesn't want to be one because dogs can't eat chocolate!

❧ Kassandra Porteous, B.F.A.
Kassie grew up in Flint, Michigan, then moved to Chicago and attended the School of the Art Institute, where she majored in design and illustration. She worked at the Anatomical Chart Company (ACC) part-time as an intern, at first, then 4 years later as a creative services manager. In the future, Kassie hopes to move to a warm climate with her husband, Michael, and their two cats, Creep and Deagle. Collecting seashells on the beach is where they will be! Which Type of Dog would she Be? A Collie, because they are loyal and reliable.